Praise for **Jorge Cruise** and *Happy Hormones, Slim Belly*™

"I'm eternally grateful to Jorge for creating a simple lifestyle plan."
— **Christiane Northrup, M.D.,**
#1 *New York Times* best-selling author of *The Wisdom of Menopause*

"Eat well without dieting or going to the gym with
Jorge's strategies for breakfast, lunch, and dinner."
— **Mehmet Oz, M.D.,**
host of *The Dr. Oz Show*

"Jorge Cruise gets it right by eliminating excessive sugar and processed carbohydrates.
His recipes and quick options make eating smart easy. I recommend them highly."
— **Andrew Weil, M.D.,**
director of the Arizona Center for Integrative Medicine,
University of Arizona, and author of *Why Our Health Matters*

"Jorge knows, as do I, that excess sugar in our diets is among
the most important factors conspiring against our waistlines and our health."
— **David Katz, M.D.,**
director and co-founder of Yale University's Prevention Research Center
and nutrition columnist for *O, The Oprah Magazine*

"This has been one of the easiest diets I have ever been on,
and I am actually losing weight—which is the best part!"
— **Linda Maze, 52**

"This plan has stopped the sugar cravings and made me feel better.
I started out thinking that I would fail like I have on every diet.
The amount of weight that I have already lost has made me extremely happy and grateful."
— **Cindy Davenport, 55**

happy hormones,
slim belly™

Other Books by
JORGE CRUISE

The 100™

Inches Off! Your Tummy™

The Aging Cure™

The Belly Fat Cure™

The Belly Fat Cure™ *Diet*

The Belly Fat Cure™ *Sugar & Carb Counter*

The Belly Fat Cure™ *Fast Track*

The Belly Fat Cure™ *Quick Meals*

Body at Home™

The 12-Second Sequence™

The 3-Hour Diet™

The 3-Hour Diet™ *Cookbook*

The 3-Hour Diet™ *for Teens*

The 3-Hour Diet™ *On-the-Go*

8 Minutes in the Morning®

8 Minutes in the Morning®*: Extra-Easy Weight Loss*

8 Minutes in the Morning®*: Flat Belly*

8 Minutes in the Morning®*: Lean Hips and Thin Thighs*

PLEASE VISIT:

Jorge Cruise: www.jorgecruise.com
Hay House USA: www.hayhouse.com®
Hay House Australia: www.hayhouse.com.au
Hay House UK: www.hayhouse.co.uk
Hay House South Africa: www.hayhouse.co.za
Hay House India: www.hayhouse.co.in

happy hormones, *slim* belly™

Over 40?
Lose 7 lbs.
the First Week
and Then 2 lbs.
Weekly—
Guaranteed

JORGE CRUISE

HAY HOUSE, INC.

Carlsbad, California • New York City
London • Sydney • Johannesburg
Vancouver • Hong Kong • New Delhi

Published and distributed in the United States by: Hay House, Inc.: www.hayhouse.com •
Published and distributed in Australia by: Hay House Australia Pty. Ltd.: www.hayhouse.com.au •
Published and distributed in the United Kingdom by: Hay House UK, Ltd.: www.hayhouse.co.uk •
Published and distributed in the Republic of South Africa by: Hay House SA (Pty), Ltd.:
www.hayhouse.co.za • *Distributed in Canada by:* Raincoast: www.raincoast.com • *Published
in India by:* Hay House Publishers India: www.hayhouse.co.in

The JorgeCruise.com, Inc., team: *Managing director:* **Oliver Stephenson**/JorgeCruise.com, Inc. •
Executive assistant: **Kristin Penne**/JorgeCruise.com, Inc.

Notice: The information given here is designed to help you make informed decisions about your body
and health. The suggestions for specific foods in this program are not intended to replace appropriate or
necessary medical care. Before starting any diet or exercise program, always see your physician. If you have
specific medical symptoms, consult your physician immediately. If any recommendations given in this program
contradict your physician's advice, be sure to consult him or her before proceeding. Mention of specific products, companies, organizations, or authorities in this book does not imply endorsement by the author or the
publisher; nor does mention of specific companies, organizations, or authorities in the book imply that they
endorse this book. The author and the publisher disclaim any liability or loss, personal or otherwise, resulting
from the procedures in this program.

Product pictures, trademarks, and trademark names are used throughout this book to describe and inform
the reader about various proprietary products that are owned by others. The presentation of such information is intended to benefit the owner of the products and trademarks and is not intended to infringe upon
trademark, copyright, or other rights; nor to imply any claim to the mark other than that made by the owner.
No endorsement of the information contained in this book has been given by the owners of such products
and trademarks, and no such endorsement is implied by the inclusion of product trademarks in this book.

The reference material in this book was compiled using a number of sources, and all information was
accurate at the time of printing. Internet addresses given in this book were accurate at the time the
book went to press.

TRADEMARKS

Happy Hormones, Slim Belly	The Belly Fat Cure	Carb Swap System
Women's Carb Cycling	Ultimate Carb Swap	12-Second Sequence
The 100	3-Hour Diet	Jorge Cruise
Sugar Calories	Body at Home	8 Minutes in the Morning

Library of Congress Control Number: 2013945811

Tradepaper ISBN: 978-1-4019-4329-5

16 15 14 13   4 3 2 1

1st edition, December 2013

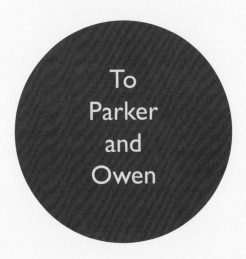

To
Parker
and
Owen

contents

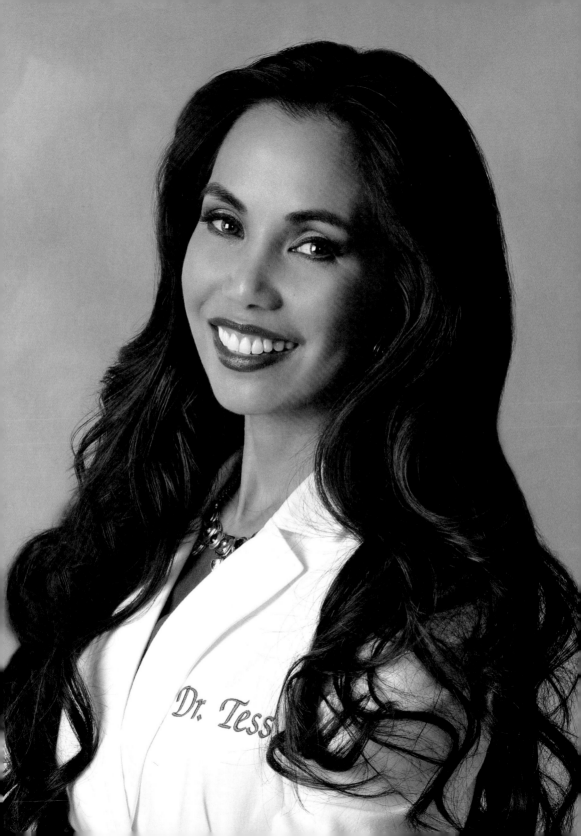

Dear Reader,

As a mother of two and a woman in my 40s, I empathize with my patients who tell me that losing weight and looking good is so much harder after they reach midlife! When my patients ask about some tips they can use to get more youthful skin and a slimmer body, I reveal a discovery many are not aware of—keeping sugar levels low to preserve collagen and maintain a healthy weight.

The latest dietary science that Jorge taught me is that carbohydrates, or "Sugar Calories," raise not only insulin but also serotonin, the feel-good neurotransmitter that helps us feel normal and balanced. The shocking truth is that women over 40 crave Sugar Calories because we are fulfilling a biological imperative to restore our lower levels of serotonin associated with aging. This revelation and awareness has made it easier for me to not be so hard on myself. I am now able to eat carbs in a way that is healthier, while still feeling happy and normal. **Jorge's brilliant concept of "Happy Days" and "Slim Days" makes it simple to create an eating plan that women will find doable— and a lifestyle they can easily stick with.**

I am always in search of the latest scientific information to help me maintain my weight and look my best. Naturally, I share what I have learned with my patients who are also searching for these answers. After discovering Jorge's Women's Carb Cycling™ program I have been able to keep my cravings at bay and my hormones balanced, helping me look and feel even more amazing! In his book *Happy Hormones, Slim Belly*™, Jorge has finally revealed the key to women's weight loss and helps all of us women around the world to look and feel as beautiful as we should.

If you are struggling with weight, affected by adverse hormonal changes, or simply feel off, this is the book that will get you on a path to great health without feeling deprived. And remember: it's not about vanity, it's about loving yourself and the skin you're in!

TESS MAURICIO, M.D.

Dr. Tess Mauricio, "America's Favorite Dermatologist," is a world-renowned board-certified dermatologist, physician trainer, and author of *California Total Beauty*. She has appeared on *The Rachael Ray Show, America's Next Top Model, The Doctors,* and *The Talk;* and has been featured in magazines around the world. For more information on Dr. Tess, please visit: www.mbeautyclinic.com.

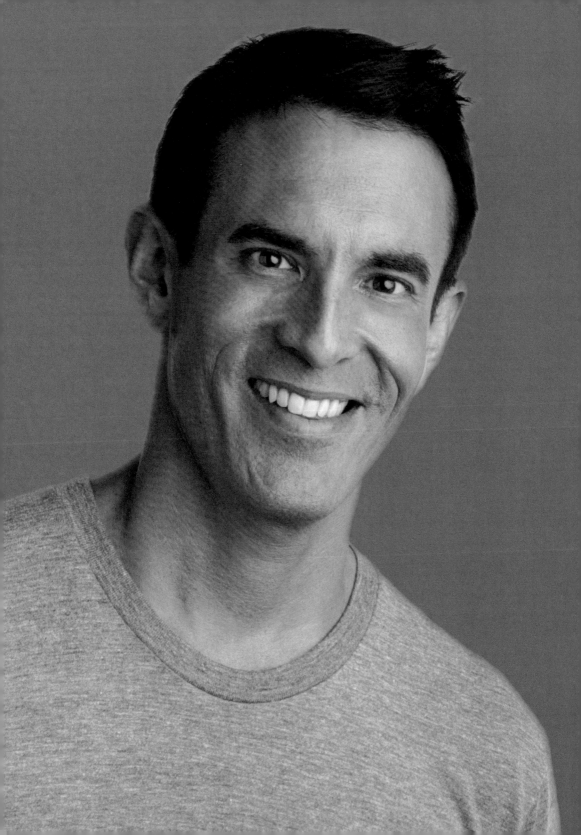

Welcome!

For any woman who has ever cut calories, or followed a starvation weight-loss program, you have an 87 percent chance of suffering from a broken metabolism, making weight loss after 40 nearly impossible. In addition, when women enter this unique stage of their life there is a biological imperative to level out imbalanced hormones with foods you thought were unhealthy for you—*until now*.

Hormonal stages that begin around age 40 and last up until age 60 initiate an ironic situation. The key to weight loss, as I have discovered with my past programs, is to keep insulin low by avoiding hidden sugars and cutting carbs. However, as breakthrough science tells us, for women over 40 there is a stronger craving for carbs due to a biological imperative to raise serotonin levels. Eating carbs triggers a complex chain of events that raises serotonin, relieving anxiety and producing happiness. (Serotonin is a critical chemical messenger that moderates mood, appetite, cravings, and impulse control.) Therefore, following the first strategy of weight loss backfires for women over 40 because it causes extreme carb and sugar cravings, but eating these foods causes weight gain. The question is: how can these two pieces work together to solve this dilemma?

The answer to fixing a broken metabolism and losing weight long-term is Women's Carb Cycling™. Guaranteed by science, this method of eating resets your insulin sensitivity, keeping you slim, while simultaneously elevating serotonin levels, which keeps you happy, energized, and free of cravings. This strategy keeps both your fat-burning engine and your motivation revved so you can lose up to 7 pounds the first week and 2 pounds weekly—guaranteed—while feeling fabulous, never deprived or hungry.

Ready to learn how you can slim down successfully, while feeling energized, inspired, and happy? You've chosen the right book! I'm thrilled to share this journey with you. Let's get started!

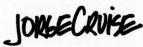

I

the irony:
How to Be Happy and Slim

It truly isn't your fault! You've been following all the rules of weight loss, just as your doctors, trainers, programs, magazine articles, and diet books have told you to—it's just that you were handed a pack of misguided advice. You don't lack willpower or possess some sort of personal weakness. There isn't anything wrong with you—what's wrong is the diet advice that has been widely spread since the 1950s.

Incredible as it might seem, most of the multimillion-dollar diets on the market are actually designed with inherent flaws that cause them to backfire. The main mistake that these diets make is telling you that the key to losing weight is to cut calories, eat a low-fat diet, and exercise more. While it's possible that the diet industry is set up to fail you so you remain forever dependent (as some conspiracy theorists posit), the mantra to "eat less and move more" is so ingrained in our society and has been around for so long that I'm not sure the folks who design most weight-loss programs even realize that their advice is misleading.

Furthermore, there's an additional problem when it comes to women over 40. Even if a weight-loss plan is on the right track, most women over 40 find that it ultimately backfires for them.

THE
IRONY

Women over 40 need to both cut Sugar Calories and add Sugar Calories (carbs) to repair their metabolism and balance out their hormones and neurotransmitters. How do you do both simultaneously? Therein lies the biggest irony no other weight-loss program has talked about, until now.

Throughout my career, and especially over the past decade, I have gained a wealth of information from my online clients at jorgecruise.com. Specifically, two critical issues have come to my attention. First, the large majority of my clients are women and, notably, most of them are over the age of 40. Second, while many of these same clients initially have great weight-loss success on my past programs, such as The 100™ (for rapid results) or The Belly Fat Cure™ (my core weight-loss plan), they would inevitably say they hit a plateau or were not able to keep the weight off in the long run. (*Note:* Both The 100™ and The Belly Fat Cure™ work successfully by counting and limiting Sugar Calories, which I will discuss further in Chapter 2.)

As I observed these women struggling, blaming themselves, and needing extra help to get back on track, I began asking myself if they needed more motivation or support in some way—or was something else going on? What was *missing?* I knew it couldn't be their fault. I know that my clients, like most women, are deeply sincere and motivated to make a change. So what else could be going on here?

That's when I turned my attention to researching scientific studies aimed at women over 40 and weight loss—I was shocked by what I discovered. The bottom line is twofold. First, previous dieting efforts by way of dramatically cutting calories make weight loss nearly impossible because they recalibrate a person's metabolism to constantly fight back. Second, when serotonin is low, it causes people to uncontrollably crave carbs (or Sugar Calories—for more information, see the box "What is a Sugar Calorie?" on the next page), and many women over 40, especially those in pre- or perimenopause, *have* just that issue going on—low serotonin. *Bingo.*

The light bulb went on: It wasn't a lack of self-control or a lack of motivation that these women were struggling with, but a natural, biological imperative to consume sugar and carbs to correct low serotonin levels. This is where I realized the incongruity: women need to cut Sugar Calories to lose weight *yet* still have Sugar Calories to keep their serotonin up, which inevitably repairs their broken metabolism.

I started talking to my clients and going through my years of notes from the women I have worked with in the past. I was blown away by my findings—if women were over 40 and dieting, they were all feeling "off" and had trouble sticking to a plan long-term. All of my research pointed to the fact that it was due to low serotonin.

Carbohydrates Are Actually Sugar!

"The basic building block of every carbohydrate is a sugar molecule,
a simple union of carbon, hydrogen, and oxygen. Starches and fibers
are essentially chains of sugar molecules . . . The digestive system handles
all carbohydrates in much the same way—it breaks them down
(or tries to break them down) into single sugar molecules, since only these
are small enough to cross into the bloodstream. It also converts most
digestible carbohydrates into glucose (also known as blood sugar),
because cells are designed to use this as a universal energy source."

— HARVARD SCHOOL OF PUBLIC HEALTH,
www.hsph.harvard.edu/nutritionsource/carbohydrates-full-story

What is a Sugar Calorie?

Any carbohydrate in a food (including all sugars) is a Sugar Calorie.
This is because all carbohydrates and sugars are broken down
into glucose (the body's sugar) at a molecular level.

It wasn't their fault, and it's not *your* fault either. All women over 40 *must* add Sugar Calories in their diet to feel good enough to eat right, even though they need to cut Sugar Calories to lose weight. This contradictory situation women find themselves in is what led me to an amazing study from researchers at the Genesis Prevention Center at the University Hospital in South Manchester, England, which helped me create the plan in this book, Women's Carb Cycling™.

These researchers noticed that when women in their study restricted what I call Sugar Calories in their diet for just two days a week, they lost nearly twice as much weight and body fat compared to women who ate an overall calorie-restricted diet (a Mediterranean-style diet with 1,500 calories per day) all seven days of the week. Another striking benefit to using this strategy can be seen in the dieters who cut Sugar Calories for two days a week: they reduced their insulin resistance by 14 to 22 percent, while the blanket calorie cutters saw only a 4 percent improvement.

Structure of Sugar and Carbohydrates

SUGAR: saccharides containing hydrogen, carbon, and oxygen

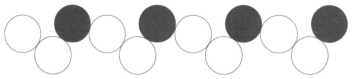

CARBOHYDRATE: polysaccharides containing long chains of hydrogen, carbon, and oxygen

What is serotonin?

Serotonin is a chemical messenger (also called a neurotransmitter) that is responsible for modulating and controlling the effects of appetite, food cravings, impulse control, motivation, and mood.

These British researchers have revealed a dieting strategy that has never before been commonly prescribed to women, but which appears to be extremely successful. The results: by cutting Sugar Calories for just two days of the week, these women were able to reset their bodies so that they were at maximum fat-burning mode and minimum fat-storing mode. Furthermore, by returning to healthy eating, which includes intermittently adding back carbs, the women were able to satisfy something that is missing on most low-calorie diets—they were able to feed their serotonin receptors.

In Chapters 2 and 3 we'll delve into the science behind serotonin (the "nirvana neurotransmitter") and the other hormones that keep your weight loss on track. For now, just know that serotonin is critical in keeping you both *happy* and *slim* for the long-term. This method of Women's Carb Cycling™ is critical because it uniquely addresses the weight gain, belly fat, mood swings, and sugar cravings caused by the wild hormonal fluctuations that women over 40 experience.

SOLVING THE PUZZLE

Now we clearly understand that the key to losing belly fat is to avoid Sugar Calories, but for women over 40, *completely* avoiding Sugar Calories inevitably leads to negative emotions, sugar cravings, and out-of-control bingeing. The overeating of Sugar Calories then leads to weight gain, belly fat, and feelings of failure.

To put it another way: The one thing you must avoid to get slim is the very thing you must have to stay slim long-term. The solution to this irony is my Women's Carb Cycling™ Plan, a way of eating based on cycling between 2 Slim Days and 5 Happy Days.

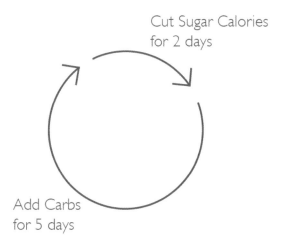

Cut Sugar Calories
for 2 days

Add Carbs
for 5 days

NEXT STEPS

Just as if I were stocking a toolbox to build a sturdy house with a strong foundation, I will make sure you are prepared with all the tools you need to know how to match your body's genetic blueprint so you can achieve lasting weight loss while feeling energized, happy, and satisfied.

In the next two chapters, I'll explain all your tools for weight-loss success in detail: the science behind getting and staying slim, and how to keep your hormones and neurotransmitters balanced so you stay happy. However, if you prefer to skip straight to your Carb Cycling Plan in Chapter 4, feel free.

In Chapter 4 I'll explain how to use the tools you've been given so you can begin your new way of eating. You'll get four weeks of meal planners and shopping lists, so you can start right away.

THE PLAN GUARANTEED BY SCIENCE FOR WOMEN OVER 40

Why do women over 40 have a stronger craving for carbs? Science has revealed that most women over 40 have a biological imperative to eat Sugar Calories to correct imbalanced hormones; however, this causes weight gain. The irony is that you must cut Sugar Calories to lose weight but you must also add Sugar Calories to keep it off long-term.

POINT 1

There is a biological impulse for women over 40 to balance hormones through Sugar Calories. Why? According to scientific research, the majority of women over 40 have lower levels of serotonin than younger women or men of any age. This has been identified in studies looking at women in perimenopause and who have higher rates of depression (depression is believed to be a disorder of *low serotonin*). Here are five examples of the many scientific studies that show this link:

A) **Around 20% of women going through perimenopause suffer depression.**

Soares CN, Taylor V. "Effects and Management of the Menopausal Transition in Women With Depression and Bipolar Disorder." *J Clin Psychiatry.* 2007;68 (suppl 9):16–21.

B) **Depressed mood is increased in women suffering hormonal fluctuations during perimenopause.**

Freeman EW, Sammel MD, Liu L, Gracia CR, Nelson DB, Hollander L. "Hormones and Menopausal Status as Predictors of Depression in Women in Transition to Menopause." *Arch Gen Psychiatry.* Jan 2004;61, no. 1:62–70.

C) **Women are twice as likely to develop depression once they enter the menopausal years, according to Harvard University researchers.**

Cohen LS, Soares CN, Vitonis AF, Otto MW, Harlow BL. "Risk for new onset of depression during the menopausal transition: the Harvard study of moods and cycles." *Arch Gen Psychiatry.* Apr 2006;63(4):385–90.

D) **Women's depressive symptoms increase during the transition from pre- to perimenopause and from peri- to postmenopause. (When estrogen plummets so does serotonin, and low levels of both are linked to depression.) During perimenopausal years, women show more depressive symptoms.**

Maartens LW, Knottnerus JA, Pop VJ. "Menopausal transition and increased depressive symptomatology: a community based prospective study." *Maturitas.* Jul 25 2002;42(3):195–200.

E) The fluctuating levels of a woman's hormones, particularly estrogen and progesterone, affect her neurotransmitter systems and may increase her vulnerability to depression and other mood disorders.

Steiner M, Dunn E, Born L. "Hormones and mood: from menarche to menopause and beyond." *J Affect Disord.* Mar 2003;74(1):67–83.

POINT 2

While cutting Sugar Calories is the key to losing weight, as said above, women over 40 have a natural craving for Sugar Calories to make up for low serotonin. Fortunately, by intermittently having carbs (Sugar Calories) and then cutting carbs, you increase insulin sensitivity, allowing you to not gain weight when you do add more of those carbs back in. Here are three major studies that have put intermittent fasting (cutting carbs or calories two days a week) to the test:

A) Intermittent fasting (cutting calories for just 2 days a week) increases insulin sensitivity.

Anson, M.R. 2003. "Intermittent fasting dissociates beneficial effects of dietary restriction on glucose metabolism and neuronal resistance to injury from calorie intake." *Proceedings of the National Academy of Sciences of the United States of America.* 100(10): 6216–6220.

B) Restricting carbs for two days a week increases insulin levels by 22% and helps women lose twice as much weight as those who diet every day of the week.

Harvie, M.N., et al. 2011. "The effects of intermittent or continuous energy restriction on weight loss and metabolic disease risk markers: a randomized trial in young overweight women." *International Journal of Obesity.* 35(5):714–727.

C) Intermittent fasting reduces blood pressure and increases insulin sensitivity. Cellular and molecular effects of intermittent fasting on the cardiovascular system and the brain are similar to those of regular physical exercise.

Mattson MP, Wan R. 2005. "Beneficial effects of intermittent fasting and caloric restriction on the cardiovascular and cerebrovascular systems." *Journal of Nutritional Biochemistry.* Mar;16(3):129–37. Review.

Therefore, you can eat carbs (Sugar Calories) to make up for lower serotonin levels and still lose weight by using the Women's Carb Cycling™ Plan, which cycles between limiting Sugar Calories and then adding them back to balance hormones and help you lose up to 7 pounds the first week and 2 pounds every week after.

WOMEN ARE NOT MEN

Did you know that the majority of dieting recommendations you hear are actually based on research with observations made solely on male subjects? Historically speaking, most scientific studies used only men as subjects because the human male is, as one expert said to me, "less complicated."

This is a popular argument: It's a hassle, some researchers say, to deal with raging hormones that fluctuate based on age and monthly cycles. Others argue that the female body is "constantly fluctuating" or "too complex" to deliver valid results in controlled studies. So, ironically, it was the very fact that women are different that was used as an excuse to exclude them from studies! While it is true that women's bodies are complex and unique, this is the exact reason that it's essential to have scientific studies that focus specifically on the female gender. And, further, to find a true working weight-loss solution, research needs to address the different life stages of women as well—but most often this isn't the case.

That said, it's not all bad news. Thanks to the National Institutes of Health instituting its Policy on the Inclusion of Women and Minorities as Subjects in Clinical Research, it is now required that women be included in clinical studies, when appropriate, in order to receive funding. Thanks to this, groundbreaking findings that address how a woman's body works on a genetic level have begun to see the light of day. It's these findings that I put into practice throughout this book to offer a solution for lasting, successful weight loss.

DIETS DON'T WORK

Most diets are a roller coaster of ups and downs, and unfortunately, there are many more ups (in pounds) than downs. According to researchers from the University of California, Los Angeles, who reviewed 31 long-term studies of diets, at least one-third to two-thirds of dieters regain more weight within four or five years than they initially lost. The study's lead author, Traci Mann, said, "We concluded most of them would have been better off not going on the diet at all. Their weight would be pretty much the same, and their bodies would not suffer the wear and tear from losing weight and gaining it all back."

In a similar study, researchers analyzed weight data of more than 14,000 people, aged 20 to 84 years, from the 1999 to 2006 National Health and Nutrition Examination Survey (NHANES). They found that only 17 percent of people who are overweight or obese are able to maintain even a 10 percent reduction in weight after a year.

Since it seems pretty apparent that diets don't work, it's even more appalling when you realize that somewhere around half of Americans are on a diet on any given day. No wonder most of us feel so burned out and frustrated about weight loss.

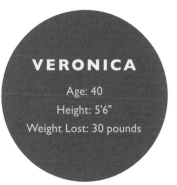

VERONICA

Age: 40
Height: 5'6"
Weight Lost: 30 pounds

I've been dieting since I was 12 years old and have never been able to keep off the weight successfully. So naturally I was a little skeptical that Jorge had found the answer, but I liked what he was saying about eating in a way that matched the life stage I was entering.

Before I started the Women's Carb Cycling™ Plan, I was achy and tired all the time, but in just one week I noticed that I felt energized and that most of my aches and pains had subsided.

BEST STRATEGY:

I used to get really bad sugar cravings in the afternoon around 3 P.M.; if I didn't give in, then at night I'd find myself bingeing on whatever carbs I could get my hands on. I've learned to save one carb snack—a piece of fruit, a couple rice cakes or cups of popcorn, or a baggie of Cheerios—for this time of day when I feel the cravings take over. Mission accomplished—the cravings have disappeared.

BIGGEST CHALLENGE:

Finding fast-food options. Because of my job's crazy hours, I eat out a lot. Here are my favorites: At Wendy's I can get the Cobb salad (just ditch the croutons on Slim Days); at In-N-Out, I order my burger "protein style," which means it's wrapped in lettuce leaves instead of a bun; and at KFC, I get the grilled chicken with a side of coleslaw.

GREATEST PAYOFF:

I used to avoid going to the grocery store because of how tired carrying in all the bags made me—now it's a breeze. The aching and swelling in my knees and feet are gone!

2

the key to a slim belly

Before we discuss anything further, it is vitally important to take a moment to acknowledge that what you've been taught about calories and weight loss is wrong. Conventional wisdom, repeated by the government and health organizations, tells us that we must cut calories to lose weight, with the philosophy that all calories are created equal. This simply isn't true. Weight gain and weight loss are fundamentally controlled only by certain foods—and only these calories count! On the other side of the calorie equation lives a multitude of foods that don't count. That's why my weight-loss mantra has become "Count only Sugar Calories!"

THE KEY TO SLIM

Fortunately for all of us, we're not going to start from ground zero. Thanks to more than ten years of research, the great success of my previous books, and more than a thousand testimonials from my successful clients, I know that I've been doing a lot of things right in this weight-loss game. Let's take a look at these keys to success: respecting insulin, making the calorie connection, and understanding the role that sugar plays in fat accumulation.

Drowning in Sugar Calories

If you're a woman who has struggled with her weight, then you probably don't need me to tell you that most diets on the market tend to fail in the long run. The majority of you have been on numerous food plans, and have probably at one time or another succeeded in losing weight—only to have it return over time.

The three diets you have probably heard the most about over the years—thanks to enormous celebrity publicity campaigns and media promotions—are Weight Watchers, Jenny Craig, and Nutrisystem. Yet I've heard from my clients for over a decade that these programs ultimately fail for them, and they regain all the weight they lost and then some. From the way these diets are promoted, it seems that hundreds of women lose weight and live happily ever after, but when you look closely at the components of these programs you can easily see where they go wrong.

First, all three diets end up being far too high in Sugar Calories, which keeps your insulin levels elevated, making you accumulate fat. In my book *The 100*™ I shared that 100 Sugar Calories a day provides the greatest amount of weight loss without the negative effects of slashing carbs (I'll elaborate further on Sugar Calories later). Unfortunately, a standard day on one of the above popular regimens ranges from 650 to more than 900 Sugar Calories! That is some serious insulin spiking at work. At this level of Sugar Calories, your body is triggered to build and add fat. Plus, these diets leave women feeling hungry and deprived—this is not the case with my plan.

Second, two out of three of the programs, Nutrisystem and Jenny Craig, require that you eat a large amount of packaged, processed foods; and many of my clients have told me that the touted ease of preparation leaves a lot to be desired. They report that the meals taste, well, *packaged,* and they find themselves staring longingly at the real food the rest of their family and friends get to eat (food that these same women oftentimes prepared themselves!) while they must eat out of little plastic containers and pouches. Plus, many women tell me that even if they do reach their desired weight on these programs, they regain the pounds quickly because they don't know what to eat once they are off the program. Even when women say they can mostly eat "real foods" on a diet, such as on Weight Watchers, they complain that the points system makes them feel too dependent and in the dark about knowing what to eat in the real world.

Finally, all of the programs ultimately function by the "calories in versus calories out" model—they cut overall calories to an average of 1,300 to 1,600 per day. The problem is that these calories are skewed far too high in Sugar Calories, so they encourage your body to accumulate and hold on to stubborn fat, and they don't satisfy hunger. In fact, many studies report that these types of diets cause you to feel hungry, deprived, and weak. On the flip side, if you eat a similar number of calories overall, but limit Sugar Calories (like you do on my plans), and cycle your carb consumption (as you'll learn to do in later chapters), you won't feel deprived, hungry, or weak. Instead, you'll lose fat while feeling energized, happy, and completely satisfied.

The bottom line: It's the quality of the food you eat, not the quantity, that matters.

OUTSMART YOUR HORMONES

If you want to be slim forever, the key is to consistently lower insulin levels in your body. Insulin is the hormone that causes your body to make fat, store fat, and hold on to fat long-term. Insulin "tells" your fat cells to hold on to the fat it has, stimulates the creation of fat, and stops the breakdown of fat to be used for energy. That's why learning how to regulate insulin is an essential part of any successful weight-loss plan.

Regulating insulin means limiting sugars from all sources because sugar, in any form, activates insulin. The logic here is that carbohydrates are broken down into glucose (your body's version of sugar) in your bloodstream, increasing your blood sugar levels, which triggers the release of insulin. Protein and fats don't elicit this response, so when you eat a meal containing carbohydrates (Sugar Calories), that meal stimulates insulin, and that insulin tells your body to burn up carbs, and to transform and store fat and protein into fat in your fat cells and liver. In other words, insulin tells your body to store glucose, to increase fat, to hang on to existing fat, to inhibit the breakdown of fat, and to burn glucose rather than fat for energy. Ultimately, all carbohydrates stimulate insulin secretion, which drives fat production and storage, leading to weight gain and obesity. This is why it is more accurate to refer to any carbohydrate as a Sugar Calorie.

The other nutrients, proteins and fats, are far more dense than Sugar Calories. They take more work by your body to digest, and they need to be broken down and then rebuilt before being transformed into glucose—and this process does not result in an elevation in insulin.

This may all seem a bit shocking because you've always heard that whole grains and fruit were a significant part of a healthy diet, but this conventional wisdom has misled you. Eating too many of these foods actually sabotages your best efforts at weight loss. I'm asking you to consider a new frame of mind about the foods you eat that is based on the way your body is designed to work. This means that you must start to view bread as a loaf of sugar, an apple as sugar, and energy bars as little rectangles of sugar. I know it is a lot to take in, but stick with me—this shift in your thinking will help you truly understand the role that these foods play in your body.

MAKE THE CALORIE CONNECTION

Let's take a closer look at calories. The truth is that the only calories that really do count and cause weight gain are the ones that trigger insulin, namely Sugar Calories. That's why I often tell my clients, "Count only Sugar Calories to successfully lose weight." Remember, all carbohydrates and sugars are broken down and "read" by your body as sugar on a molecular level, so I believe it is more accurate to refer to all carbohydrates and sugars as Sugar Calories. On the other hand, proteins, healthy fats, and low-sugar vegetables can be called "Freebie Foods" because they liberate fat from your body and cause weight loss. Since Sugar Calories are the only calories that matter when it comes to losing weight, knowing how to limit and regulate them is the secret to successful weight loss. The tricky part comes in for women, especially women over 40, because it isn't as simple as just cutting all Sugar Calories from the diet. The key to being slim is keeping Sugar Calories in their place, and I'll teach you how to do this in the following chapters.

WHAT ARE FREEBIE FOODS?

Freebie Foods are healthy proteins, fats, and vegetables
that are so low in Sugar Calories and so high in nutrients
that they needn't be tracked. As long as you consume these foods
in reasonable portions as part of a healthy diet, you don't
need to worry about counting the calories in Freebie Foods
because they actually work to liberate fat, not to store it on your body.
In Chapter 7 you'll find extensive lists of
Freebie Foods that will make eating to stay slim
and happy an effortless part of the rest of your life.

UNDERSTAND THE SINS OF SUGAR

I hold steady to the ever-growing body of evidence that sugars of all types are addictive and, in excessive quantities, toxic to the human body—they cause weight gain, prevent weight loss, and create disease. This includes all sources of sugars and carbohydrates.

We humans are not made to consume the amounts of sugars that we do today—which is why, before the introduction and mass production of refined sugars and flours in the 1700s, we didn't struggle with obesity the way we do today. In fact, for 99.5 percent of our genetic history as human beings we were hunter-gatherers who consumed diets that were primarily meat, leafy greens, seeds, and nuts; with the only sugars coming from the occasional fruits that were in season, and honey when it could be found. Consider this: the amount of sugars (this includes table sugar made from sugarcane and beets, and corn sweeteners—notably high-fructose corn syrup, aka HFCS) that each person eats per day has increased by 43 pounds, or 39 percent, from 1950–59 to 2000. In 2000, each American consumed an average of 152 pounds of sugar—that's 52 teaspoonfuls, or 6.5 servings of Coke—per person per

BELINDA

Age: 56
Height: 5'5"
Weight Lost: 22 pounds

I've been in menopause for more than a year now, so I wasn't sure that this diet would work for me. But since I suffer from low moods and find myself fighting uncontrollable cravings for ice cream at home and the bread basket at restaurants, I thought Jorge's plan might be a good one for me.

BEST STRATEGY:
Keeping the on-the-go options on hand. I used my phone to take pictures of each page with these fast options so that I could "carry" them with me everywhere I went.

BIGGEST CHALLENGE:
For me, the weight came off slowly at first. With just a three-pound weight loss at the end of the first week I started to get discouraged, but then I read about tracking the inches I was losing. I was thrilled to see that I was losing inches steadily, and my clothes quickly fit better and got loose long before the scale said anything.

GREATEST PAYOFF:
My low moods have vanished along with my cravings for sweets and bread. Cutting out Sugar Calories for just two days a week is a breeze, and often I find that I can follow the Extra-Slim Plan with no issues. The best compliment I've heard? My four-year-old granddaughter saying to her friend, "My grandma has so much energy, she makes me tired at the playground."

day! Interestingly, our history of weight gain and obesity follows the same trajectory as our history of increased sugar consumption.

Often HFCS is called out as the supreme villain of sugar, but I want to point out that *all* sugars are really composed of extremely similar, and destructive, components—specifically, fructose. While HFCS is composed of 55 percent fructose and 45 percent glucose, most other sugars, including table sugar, are made of a 50/50 ratio. The percentage difference is so minuscule that really all sugars should get the supervillain label, not just corn sweeteners such as HFCS.

Robert Lustig, a pediatric endocrinologist and professor at the University of California, San Francisco, and world-renowned sugar expert, earned fame because of his arguments about fructose's adverse effects on humans. On May 26, 2009, he delivered a lecture called "Sugar: The Bitter Truth," which was posted on the UCTV channel on YouTube the following July and went "viral" with over 3 million views at the time of this writing. It's incredibly informative and worth watching; you can see it at http://youtu.be/dBnniua6-oM.

The research on caloric sweeteners and obesity is well known, and not many experts argue the strong link between excess fat on the body and excess sugar in the diet. What you need to know is that too much sugar acts as a toxin in your body. The fructose in sugar can't be processed through the bloodstream like other nutrients. Instead, it goes to the liver (where toxins are handled) where it is broken down into dangerous free radicals as well as a form of fat called triglycerides, which can cause liver damage and the buildup of plaque in artery walls. High fructose intake can also cause insulin resistance. The other half of sugars—the glucose portion—spikes your insulin and tells your body to store and to hang on to fat. It's a double whammy that is at the core of our obesity epidemic. To make matters even worse, because of the chemical composition of liquid sugars (most often high-fructose corn syrup), your brain doesn't register it, according to a new study published in *The Journal of the American Medical Association*. That means that when you consume high-sugar drinks, your body doesn't even notice it, and it makes you hungrier, so you consume far more food over the course of the day.

After sugars, highly refined carbs are next in line as the calories that cause fat to accumulate on your body, because they are processed almost exactly the same way sugar is. Carbs don't have the fructose component, so your liver isn't taxed, but their glucose still spikes your insulin as dramatically and instantly as sugar does, which tells your body to create and store fat. This is why, regardless of whether a food is a carb or a sugar, to your body it registers as a Sugar Calorie, and Sugar Calories equal fat accumulation and weight gain.

Now that we've discussed the most highly refined Sugar Calories, what about whole grains? While we have been educated that they are an essential part of any healthy diet, this is misleading because whole grains are still made up of a great amount of insulin-raising Sugar Calories. Many will argue that a piece of whole-wheat bread will break down more slowly than a soda, and they are right; but the amount of insulin that will be secreted can be similar.

The same reasoning about whole grains can be applied to fruits—even though there are great benefits from vitamins and nutrients, the amount of sugar that fruit can contain may sabotage your weight loss by stimulating your appetite and further cravings for sugar. However, the jury is still out on fruit. Some agencies and experts say that the sugar and carbs in fruit don't count because they are offset by the fiber and water content, while others say that it can still alter weight loss. Therefore, I suggest keeping fruit servings to no more than two a day. It's important to keep in mind that these, along with many other "healthy" foods, must be viewed as Sugar Calories, and they need to be tracked for successful weight loss.

THE IMPORTANCE OF BALANCED EATING

One of the reasons why we need to be so careful about tracking Sugar Calories today is because most of us have followed flawed diets, and these past efforts have caused us to have chronically elevated insulin as well as a broken metabolism. Consider for a moment the fact that, for at least ten generations, we've been eating a diet that consists of far too many Sugar Calories. This way of eating is what caused the obesity epidemic and the whopping spike in diabetes and other disorders.

Even more shocking is the fact that we were likely set up to have chronically elevated insulin while we were still in our mother's belly. Think about it: if a woman is eating a diet high in Sugar Calories, that means that her pancreas (where insulin is produced) is consistently pumping out high levels of insulin. A mother's pancreas plays a key role in the nutrition of the developing infant because it mediates the transport of nutrition to the fetus, including blood sugar. High blood sugar levels in a pregnant woman causes the baby's own insulin levels to go up as a result, leading to increased fat and a higher birth weight. The result is an infant born already "addicted" to high levels of Sugar Calories. This sets us up from birth to crave Sugar Calories and store more fat than we should.

This severe imbalance, caused by a diet of too many Sugar Calories that started in our childhoods and even possibly in the womb, requires that we implement a plan that strictly limits even the Sugar Calories that might be the healthiest (fruits and whole grains). Over time, you may become more insulin sensitive and able to add back in some fruit and whole grains. The good news is that by using Carb Cycling you can reverse the effects of chronically elevated insulin levels and quickly become more insulin sensitive, which reduces the harmful effects of carbs and sugars—and also helps reduce your cravings for them.

Of all the things I've learned about putting together a food plan that will guarantee weight-loss success, the most essential to remember is that you must have the right balance of overall nutrients that matches your biological needs. However, balanced doesn't mean equal amounts of each nutrient—it means meeting the right levels of each nutrient as required by your individual body, which is determined by your body's basic needs (being human), your gender (being female), and your age (over 40).

New research from *The Journal of the American Medical Association* brings this "being human" part home by comparing a low-fat, a low-carb, and a low-sugar diet. The Harvard researchers found that the most successful diet is low in sugars. Here's the rub: humans need a diet that keeps insulin low enough (by strictly limiting Sugar Calories) so that the body can let go of excess weight, while women need to eat the right amount and kinds of Sugar Calories at the right time to keep hormones balanced and cravings in check. It is not so much the high number of overall calories as it is the overeating of Sugar Calories that perpetuates the obesity epidemic—and so to the next point.

Cutting overall calories and eating a diet low in fat doesn't actually result in lasting weight loss and has caused many metabolisms to slow down dramatically, even though that's the advice you've been given from government health officials, the medical community, and obesity experts for more than 60 years. In a 2002 review of low-fat and calorie-restricted diets (also appropriately referred to as semi-starvation diets), researchers from the Cochrane Collaboration concluded that "fat-restricted diets are no better than calorie-restricted diets in achieving long-term weight loss in overweight or obese people." Study after study finds that cutting calories almost always results in a regain of any weight lost.

Despite these convincing results, nearly every major health agency—including the American Heart Association, the American Medical Association, the American College of Sports Medicine, the National Institutes of Health, the Institute of Medicine, the World Health Organization, the United States Department of Health and Human Services, and the United States Department of Agriculture—still tells us that cutting calories is the way to lose weight. The reality is that this blanket method of cutting calories throws off your hormonal balance by lowering hormones and neurotransmitters that prevent overeating, including serotonin. For example, Oxford University researchers found that just three weeks on a low-calorie diet significantly reduces tryptophan, an amino acid that is necessary for the production of serotonin (more on this in the next chapter)—and the effect of tryptophan depletion was much more severe in women than in men.

As we'll explore further in the next section, it's this blatant disregard of your sensitivity to these

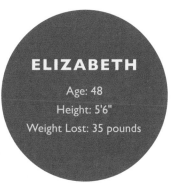

ELIZABETH

Age: 48
Height: 5'6"
Weight Lost: 35 pounds

Being a nurse, a Ph.D. student, a wife, and a mother to three teens had caused me to put my weight-loss goals on hold for a long time. I used the excuse that I just didn't have time, and that I would deal with the excess pounds after my life settled down. All that changed when I recently caught my reflection in the mirror and didn't recognize the heavy woman staring back.

BEST STRATEGY:

Learning to modify the program to fit my needs, specifically by finding ways to be more time efficient. For example, I bought frozen spinach, asparagus, and sweet potatoes, and used them in place of the fresh ones called for in recipes. This saved time and money.

BIGGEST CHALLENGE:

Leaving the house without my food for the day. I quickly learned that convenience stores such as 7-Eleven now carry great snack choices, such as string cheese, nuts, and even boiled eggs. With these options I could always make it to my next meal.

GREATEST PAYOFF:

Besides all the great comments, I loved that my family enjoyed the meals as much as I did. I didn't have to do any extra cooking. In fact, my husband loves the lasagna cups so much that he asked me to make them for the Sunday-school class he teaches. My dad, who has type 2 diabetes, liked the food so much that he decided to try the diet with me. He's lost 33 pounds, and his waist went from 42 to 36 inches!

shifts in your chemical balance that sets you up to fail. The key to successful weight loss and optimal health is to not only limit Sugar Calories but also, for women over 40, to incorporate a new method of eating that is designed specifically for your hormonal stage—and that's what we're going to do here.

The bottom line on the faulty "calories in versus calories out" philosophy of weight loss is that our bodies don't work quite so simply—we can't just fill and empty our proverbial gas tanks. Every time we eat a food it communicates something to our bodies, and our bodies respond based on the food's components to tell it where to go. So the old adage "You are what you eat" needs a minor tweak—as Eric Westman, director of the Duke University Lifestyle Medicine Clinic, likes to say, "You are what your body does with what you eat." If you are eating mostly foods that don't spike insulin, and the right amount of healthy Sugar Calories, then you'll lose weight because you'll be eating in a biologically balanced way—and it won't feel like deprivation, starvation, or punishment.

A WORD ABOUT EXERCISE

If you are thinking of hitting the "calories in versus calories out" theory of weight loss from the other end, by trying to lose weight by burning it off via exercise, forget it—that doesn't work either. This doesn't mean that exercise is not an important component in our quest for weight loss, but its role is more suited to be an essential support tool rather than our main strategy. (See Chapter 8 for my tips on how you can use and enjoy fitness as part of your weight-loss plan.) Just know that exercise on its own won't cause lasting weight loss because our bodies work hard to replace any calories we burn off during a workout. In the end it is all about our hormones.

WHAT WAS MISSING

While I believe I've made great strides in showing people how to successfully and sustainably lose weight, it has recently come to my attention that I wasn't addressing the needs of a large percentage of my clients. My past books addressed the latest diet research by identifying Sugar Calories and advocating limits on sugar and carbs in order to regulate levels of the hormone insulin, which controls fat storage. This strategy does work for weight loss, but I found a snag for women over 40. These clients were losing weight, and lots of it, but I started hearing concerns about not being able to stick with the plan because uncontrollable sugar cravings and fluctuating mood swings would surface and throw these women off track. Because I believe in the wisdom of the human body, I suspected that this glitch was due to some part of my eating plan not being in sync with what was going on for women in this age range—40 to 60—on a biological level.

This revelation that women needed something different prompted me to go on a journey to reanalyze my diet philosophy, and to review past and current research on weight loss and women. And I'll be forever indebted, because digging through the research led me to groundbreaking findings that explain the missing link for women age 40 to 60 who are trying to lose weight.

I'm sure you've heard the quote, "The only thing constant in life is change." Well, that's certainly true of the way that scientific research continually reveals findings that change our worldview and eventually how we do things. This is something I try to embrace, even when it means revising and updating what I've said and done in the past. Ultimately, I know that the best way to continue offering successful strategies for lasting weight loss is to always be open and honest about ways we can improve our methods. And while my core philosophy (to count only Sugar Calories) is still accurate, how this counting is applied for women over 40 takes some finesse.

IT'S NOT JUST FOR WOMEN OVER 40

The unique life stage I address in this book is the 15- to 20-year span that ranges from around age 40 to 55 or 60, but that doesn't mean that the plan outlined here won't work for you if you fall out of this age range. Whether you are under age 40 or over 60, the plan outlined in this book will also help you lose weight effectively.

For women under 40: Even though most women in this age range haven't begun to experience the hormonal fluctuations related to perimenopause, all women follow a more or less regular monthly hormonal cycle. During your menstrual cycle, certain chemical messengers increase, while others decrease—these changes affect how you relate to food. Happy Hormones, Slim Belly™ is designed to address these issues. Just before ovulation, many women experience extreme cravings for sugars and carbs, and the design of this program addresses these beautifully.
(In Chapter 4 you'll learn how to apply the diet to your unique stage of life.)

For women over 40: Starting at around age 40 many women begin to experience perimenopause, which is fluctuations in hormones and neurotransmitters that will eventually lead to menopause. Happy Hormones, Slim Belly™ is designed to directly address these issues. (Please see Chapter 3 for the full explanation.)

For women over 60: After menopause (defined as a lack of menstruation for at least 12 months), a woman's hormones and neurotransmitters level out, but they run at a slightly lower overall level. The Happy Hormones, Slim Belly™ way of eating optimizes your system so that the chemicals related to weight loss run smoothly and keep you feeling your best.
(Turn to Chapter 4 for suggestions on how to eat for this stage of life.)

THE NEXT STEPS

Now you are equipped and educated to lose that excess weight—you'll just limit Sugar Calories (all carbs and sugars), right? For men and some women under 40 this may be an easy task, but for the majority of women over age 40 things get a little trickier.

Starting at around age 40 until around age 60, most women undergo a series of chemical changes that affect the hormones and neurotransmitters that are intimately linked to emotions, weight gain, and weight loss. If you are in this category, then you actually require some of the right Sugar Calories, used in the correct way, to successfully lose weight. And herein lies the puzzle: how can women over 40 avoid Sugar Calories *and* include Sugar Calories to see successful long-term weight loss?

The answers can be found on the following pages.

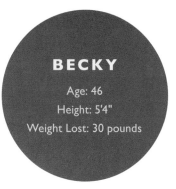

BECKY

Age: 46
Height: 5'4"
Weight Lost: 30 pounds

My weight was fine until I turned 40, then the numbers on the scale started to creep up. I started cutting back on calories, but that didn't work. My moods seemed more erratic, and I found myself often eating sweets to soothe my bummed-out emotions. By the time I was 45 I was 30 pounds overweight. While searching for solutions online I came across Jorge's website and read about a better strategy for women over 40. Not counting calories scared me, but since it wasn't working for me I decided to give HHSB a try. I dropped 8 pounds the first week!

BEST STRATEGY:

Getting educated. I really appreciate all the information that Jorge provides on how the human body works, and how we can meet its needs on a biological level. Understanding how insulin works, and addressing my needs for serotonin, really helps me stick to this new way of eating.

BIGGEST CHALLENGE:

Sugar cravings. I used to have serious late-afternoon carb cravings. If I stopped by a coffee bar, just looking at the pastries would put me in a panic. I'd try to satisfy these cravings with diet sodas or Splenda-sweetened syrups in my coffee. Often I'd still end up giving in and buying a cookie or some potato chips. After I started Jorge's diet I noticed that I no longer missed sweeteners, artificial or not, and refined carbs.

GREATEST PAYOFF:

Deep sleep. Before I lost this weight I would toss and turn at night. I could never get comfortable because my PJs would bunch up and pull on my fat. Now when I get into bed I'm so comfortable that I quickly drift away. I also notice that I wake up feeling refreshed and energized.

3

the key to
happy hormones

To illustrate how the weight-loss world for women has been set up, let me relate to you my shower problem. Honestly, cleaning the shower can be a dreadful task! Thankfully, I recently discovered an "automatic shower cleaner" on TV, which promises to do all the work for you and deliver "instant" results. I ordered it right away, but I was pretty disappointed when it arrived. This shower cleaner is really just a sprayer with a battery, and when I read the instructions carefully it said that it will take three months of daily use to have the promised sparkling shower. Who has time to wait that long for a clean shower? It really wasn't the product I was hoping for, and the old adage "When something sounds too good to be true—it probably is" comes to mind.

The point is that, like my shower gadget, most diets make big promises, but they don't deliver. Most diets require that you cut overall calories and be semi-starved in order to lose weight, only for you to regain those pounds when you inevitably can't stick to the unrealistic plan. Happy Hormones, Slim Belly™ is not a quick fix, but it does deliver big results without you ever feeling deprived. In the previous chapter I told you how to get the *slim* part down, by cutting Sugar Calories; now we need to turn to the *happy*.

The real problem is that most diets don't address how women over 40 are designed from the inside out. Instead, they are all variations on the same calorie-cutting theme—whether they come in pretty prepared packages, require counting points, or involve taking supplements. What's worse is that these diets actually lead to failure, not success. Not only do they fail to deliver lasting weight loss, they don't address your critical need for the feel-good neurotransmitter, serotonin.

If, instead of investing in a quick-fix cleaning gadget, you were to vigorously scrub the shower with the right cleaner, you would quickly see results; elbow grease is designed to match what a dirty shower needs. A good scrubbing with the right cleaner is the most effective way to get the results you want—a squeaky-clean shower. This is what the Happy Hormones, Slim Belly™ way of eating will deliver. The plan that I propose is most effective because it is designed to match how your body works on a biological level for the stage of life you are currently in. That's what the breakthrough science has delivered and what I want to share with you. Happy Hormones, Slim Belly™ is an effortless, delicious way to lose up to 7 pounds the first week and 2 pounds every week after with a large smile on your face.

The rest of this chapter will give you a glimpse into the missing link—the *happy*—that women need to make weight loss last long-term.

ADDRESSING THE HAPPY HORMONES

All of the rules for weight loss that I outlined in the previous chapter have helped hundreds of men and women lose weight and keep it off effortlessly and enjoyably. So why wasn't this strategy working consistently for my female clients who were over the age of 40? Why were so many of them e-mailing me and messaging me at jorgecruise.com to tell me that they couldn't stay on the plan when it cut out too many Sugar Calories? It was always a similar story: after a set number of days—which varied from woman to woman—I'd hear about mood swings and cravings for sugar that built up until they got to be too much. The best-laid intentions would crash, and a sugar binge would follow.

This caused insulin spikes, regained weight, and feelings of failure, which would then lead to a repetitive cycle of overeating. I knew there had to be something going on at a biological level that was linking negative emotions to sugar cravings and binges, and that's when I put on my research hat and discovered the missing link for women over 40.

In this chapter we'll take a close look at how two chemical messengers, the neurotransmitter serotonin and the hormone insulin, work to influence your moods, thoughts about food, impulse control, and appetite triggers. We'll also explore the latest scientific research that directly addresses women and all their complex and unique needs when it comes to losing weight successfully. You'll learn what it takes to work with your body so that it effortlessly lets go of excess weight, while simultaneously keeping you feeling your best. With my strategy, you will overcome any challenge and continue to lose fat and maintain your weight loss forever.

THE SECRET OF SEROTONIN

Serotonin levels determine factors such as your mood, food cravings, appetite, and impulse control. If a diet doesn't address these events, and most don't, then your long-term weight-loss success is blocked.

The reality is that just about every diet out there can deliver short-term results, but very few succeed in delivering sustainable success without tremendous sacrifice. Other diets also don't address the fundamental fact that from ages 40 to 60, women undergo dramatic chemical changes that cause them to feel blue and drained and to have mood swings that affect eating behaviors. There is a cascading effect of changing hormone and neurotransmitter levels and changing behaviors.

By incorporating these essential facts and applying strategies that balance hormones and boost serotonin, I've been able to design a way of eating that truly provides lasting weight loss for women over 40. In the next chapter I'll explain how to get results with Happy Hormones, Slim Belly™, but first I want to share with you three factors that really drive the "happy" in this program:

1. Dietary needs based on your age. What happens to a woman shortly after she turns 40 is a major change in hormonal balance. My mentor Christiane Northrup, a leading women's health expert, likes to say that this phase of life, perimenopause (the years leading up to menopause), is akin to puberty in reverse. Hormones that had followed a relatively normal cyclical nature go haywire, just like they did when you were a teenager. The difference here is that, instead of being on the incline, certain chemical messengers are decreasing—and many of these hormones and neurotransmitters affect your appetite, mood, and impulse control (see "The Skinny on Hormones" on page 32). **Knowing how to eat in a way that helps balance out these emotional fluctuations, while also controlling for your body's physical ability to burn fat, is essential.**

These hormonal changes are a somewhat modern phenomenon because prehistoric women often didn't live long enough to experience perimenopause or menopause (the average Stone Age life of a woman was around 40 years of age, not the 80 that it is today). So it made sense that our female predecessors were able sustain their health by continuing to eat mostly protein and fat, with very little carbs and hardly any sugar. In the next chapter, I'll explain how fat and protein are still good, but we need to incorporate some different strategies for including the right sort of Sugar Calories, in the right amounts, at the right time, to keep your moods fueling your motivation for weight loss.

The other issue is that, as a modern woman, you need a way of eating that taps your ancestral roots without requiring you to go on hunting excursions or forage for food in the forest. I propose a modern spin that matches your genetic blueprint and honors your ancestry. In the following chapters I'll teach you how to eat this way and what activities you can do to maximize the hormones and neurotransmitters that keep you feeling your best, which in turn keeps you on track and losing weight effortlessly.

2. Dietary needs based on your gender. Men and women have similar levels of serotonin, assuming both are healthy and not undergoing any hormonal fluctuations. However, regardless of health, women always make serotonin at a much slower rate, according to Canadian researchers at McGill University. In men, the investigators found, serotonin is made at a rate that is 52 percent faster than in women. This means that when women's serotonin levels are low due to stress, depression, or not eating the right balance of proteins and carbs (all of which lower serotonin), they can't replenish it to a healthy level fast enough. The exact mechanism still isn't understood, but scientific research suggests that women are more likely than men to suffer serotonin-related disorders such as depression, anxiety, eating disorders, migraines, seasonal affective disorder, fibromyalgia, and irritable bowel syndrome. This slower action at making serotonin has also been replicated in studies done by experts in the Netherlands. Add this handicap of not being able to make serotonin fast enough to a diet of too many Sugar Calories and not enough protein or fat, and the burden of low serotonin is multiplied.

I'm not going to tell you that I know what it's like to be a woman; however, I do empathize with my clients. Many of you, I am sure, have had children, suffer or have suffered from PMS, and are now experiencing the effects of perimenopause or menopause—all things I can understand, but can never truly experience. If you're over 40, it's likely that the first signs of perimenopause, the precursor to menopause, have begun and will continue for the next 10 to 15 years until you are in full menopause. Your serotonin levels may be low because of your life stage, and all these things influence your mood and your ability to eat healthfully.

These experiences change the chemical bath of hormones and neurotransmitters that tell your body what to do and how to feel. On top of that, these same hormones and neurotransmitters fluctuate on a daily, monthly, and seasonal cycle as well—regardless of your age. In addition, dips or spikes in chemical messengers seem to affect women more dramatically than men, according to scientific studies. And even if you took away all the cycles women go through, they still have different hormone levels in their bodies than men do—this is the beautiful and unique design of the female body, which equips women to carry babies.

There's nothing wrong with any of the things above—what's wrong is that a world of advice has been created and given using a template that was made for men, which doesn't respect how a woman's body functions—that's what I intend to remedy in this book. I believe that knowledge is power. Rather than feel a victim to your body or overwhelmed by what you've read so far, you can use the information and tools in this book to know how to work with your female body to make weight loss effortless while feeling your best.

While there are certainly variations, men have a steadier level and much more stable overall pattern of hormones than women; this makes them "easier" to study, so that's been the default in scientific studies. There's less to take into account over the course of a research trial—no periods to count, or who's in menopause, and so on—men are just men. The outcomes tend to be nice and neat. The problem of course is that the results of such studies are then generalized to all human beings—despite the fact that male answers don't work for female needs.

The accepted status quo, the old theory of calorie expenditure, dictates that we can generalize the amount of calories your body uses per day to the amount of calories you should consume. But this theory undermines the vast uniqueness in gender, not to mention the hormonal stage you are in. Our dietary model needs a serious update.

3. Dietary needs based on your biological drive for carbohydrates. Because men tend to have more balanced hormones and neurotransmitters, most men can cut Sugar Calories out of their diet without experiencing the level of serotonin depletion that women do. Remember that men make serotonin 52 percent faster than women. Women, on the other hand, can't keep serotonin levels high enough when they cut out Sugar Calories, and living without any Sugar Calories is one of the reasons that women report carb and sugar cravings, and emotional or out-of-control eating.

Research shows that low serotonin causes cravings that can only be denied for so long. Here's how it works: If a woman eats a diet that cuts all carbs and sugars, it brings her insulin levels way down, and while this is good for trimming fat, it also depletes serotonin stores. When your body detects this depletion of serotonin, it sends out triggers that cause you to have insatiable cravings for sugar. When you eat foods rich in carbohydrates and sugar, it makes your blood sugar levels rise, stimulating insulin production. Insulin speeds up the absorption of most amino acids, except for tryptophan, the precursor to serotonin. This makes it so that there is more tryptophan available for your body to convert into serotonin. The remedy is eating the right Sugar Calories, in the right amounts, at the right times to keep your insulin/serotonin relationship optimal so that you eliminate cravings and are able to stick to your weight-loss plan. In the next chapter, you'll get a full detailed plan to fit this new understanding into your life.

CURB 90% OF CARB CRAVINGS WITH VERBAL MANTRAS

Thinking positively changes your body's chemistry and eliminates cravings for Sugar Calories. Using affirmations/mantras is a powerful and effective way of doing this. Affirmations, also known as mantras, are "I" statements that you say out loud or in your mind to enhance a positive outlook and self-empowerment.

HOW IT WORKS:

When you think a negative thought, such as *I can't do it,* you release stress hormones, including cortisol and norepinephrine. When you think a happy thought, such as *I can do it,* you release feel-good neurotransmitters, such as endorphins and serotonin. It really is that fast and simple.

THE SCIENCE:

In one study by the National Institutes of Mental Health, researchers found that a particular area of the brain becomes activated when people focus on future positive events. The people lost their optimism, and showed decreased activity in that area of their brains, when their brains were deprived of serotonin. Thinking optimistically stimulates serotonin production; and among the many effects of serotonin is that it reduces cravings for Sugar Calories and enhances motivation.

Repetitive thoughts are like the deep groove a car makes driving down a dirt road, over and over. The more you think a thought, the more that related chemicals are stimulated and released.

WHAT YOU CAN DO:

Make daily affirmations part of your life to increase your serotonin, improve motivation, and eliminate cravings for Sugar Calories. For more information, and to view the daily serotonin-stimulating mantras that I've created, please visit: HappyHormonesSlimBelly.com.

THE SKINNY ON HORMONES

Both hormones and neurotransmitters are the chemical messengers secreted from your brain that are largely responsible for your behaviors, emotions, and attitudes. These chemical messengers work to maintain emotional, physical, and mental equilibrium in your body. Whenever something is out of balance—you feel overly stressed, angry, or fearful—your body responds by releasing chemicals that cause you to have an urge to do something to fix the imbalance. For example, if you find yourself craving Sugar Calories, it is often due to one of the just mentioned emotions, which usually means that the neurotransmitter serotonin is low. Eating Sugar Calories will raise serotonin. Your body doesn't know that this might not be the healthiest fix; it only knows that there is an imbalance, and the goal is to return to a balanced state.

There are so many similarities between hormones and neurotransmitters that they are often referred to interchangeably, but they are different. Most notably, hormones are released by the endocrine system into the bloodstream or extracellular fluid, while neurotransmitters are transmitted across nerve cells through electrical impulses.

What Are Neurotransmitters?

Neurotransmitters are chemical messengers that transmit information about many things including mood, appetite, cravings, impulse control, and libido, to name a few. These "messages" are nerve impulses, which are transmitted from one nerve cell to another cell (this can be a nerve, muscle, or organ cell). Many neurotransmitters regulate how you feel throughout your day. As it relates to weight gain, when there is a drop in certain neurotransmitters, it will affect your mood (which leads to emotional eating) and cause you to have a lower level of impulse control, an increased appetite, and cravings for certain foods (carbohydrates and sugars). Serotonin is the main neurotransmitter related to overeating, eating the wrong foods, and weight gain. Other neurotransmitters also related to food and mood are endorphins and dopamine.

What Are Hormones?

Hormones are chemical messengers that are secreted into the bloodstream. These chemicals regulate every activity of daily living, including controlling reproduction; regulating the growth and development of all cells; maintaining the body's internal environment (temperature, hydration); and the regulation of energy production, utilization, and storage (what we do with the food we eat). When it comes to storing and burning fat, the main hormone is insulin. When it comes to emotional eating and craving carbs, estrogen and progesterone play a critical role. Not surprisingly, these are the two hormones that change the most dramatically in women over 40.

To make matters more confusing, hormones and neurotransmitters are almost always intrinsically linked. For example, serotonin, which is a neurotransmitter, needs insulin to boost its level in the brain. There are numerous hormones and neurotransmitters in the human body, but for the purposes of this book we'll focus on those that are most intimately related to women and weight loss.

Here is a quick primer on the main hormones and neurotransmitters that are intimately linked to appetite, hunger, fat storage, emotional eating, and impulse control. While I may briefly discuss others throughout the book, the following are the hormones and neurotransmitters I'll refer to often because they are most involved in keeping you Slim and Happy.

Neurotransmitters to Remember

— *Serotonin:* This is the master neurotransmitter in the body; it modulates and controls the effects of almost all other neurotransmitters. Serotonin brings feelings of calm, happiness, peace, and satisfaction. This in turn affects your mood, impulse control, appetite, digestion, and food cravings.

— *Endorphins:* These neurotransmitters are the body's natural opiates. They act to increase feelings of pleasure. These chemicals have been shown to increase during drug use, sex, exercise, and by consuming sugars.

— *Dopamine:* This is one of those chemicals that can act as both a hormone and a neurotransmitter. Dopamine is related to the reward center in your brain. It is triggered by alcohol, drugs, and sugar.

While all these neurotransmitters are stimulated by Sugar Calories, they can also be increased by sunshine, laughter, and exercise.

Hormones to Remember

— *Insulin:* This is the master hormone in the body because it tells your body how to store and use all the fuel that comes into your system. Insulin is what drives fat into your fat cells, but it also is involved in shuttling tryptophan, the amino acid that is needed to make serotonin, into the brain. So for weight loss, you want to keep this hormone low, but for happiness, you need to keep it high.

— *Estrogen:* This and progesterone are the main female hormones that begin to fluctuate wildly during your perimenopausal years. After age 40, estrogen begins to surge and dip at varying rates, which can affect your mood, sleep habits, energy levels, and serotonin levels. Estrogen helps produce more receptor sites for serotonin in the brain, so when estrogen dips, so does serotonin.

— *Progesterone:* This is the first hormone that dips dramatically in your perimenopausal years. Not surprisingly, low progesterone has been linked to low serotonin levels. Low levels of this hormone can bring on hot flashes, insomnia, and mood swings.

I suspect that many of you already know that diets don't work from your own failed experiences. But now you know that it isn't your fault. You have been trying to follow all the rules as they have been laid out for you, and you have been misguided because the advice for losing weight is inherently designed to throw you off track. Now you know that there are specific factors that cause diets to not work for women over 40, and I've told you about the missing piece—having a diet that supports your unique chemical fluctuations that start to change after age 40.

THE CYCLE OF YOUR CHANGING BODY

I've already given you an overview of the way your body relates to its world and to itself, and how it begins to undergo a dramatic change starting as early as age 35 and lasting as long as age 60. Part of this "adolescence in reverse" is a natural decline in the hormones that support egg production for your reproductive years—estrogen and progesterone. But this is no smooth sled ride down the side of a snowy knoll. Instead, the perimenopausal years (the years leading up to menopause) are akin to skiing the steep, jagged side of a mountain on an experts-only "Black Diamond" trail.

The thing to remember as I discuss the rather technical-sounding hormones and neurotransmitters of the body is that they are all intimately related to one another. Each time one of these chemicals is released in your body, a cascading action takes place that influences the other chemicals in your body. For example, when insulin is elevated it increases the production of serotonin in your brain. When estrogen decreases it lowers insulin sensitivity, which causes a craving for Sugar Calories—and it goes on and on. There is more, but I'll hold back on the "Biology 301" details. Just remember that each and every rule of Happy Hormones, Slim Belly™ is made to optimize the levels of your body's chemicals (hormones and neurotransmitters) to induce weight loss that lasts.

There are quite a few hormonal fluctuations during perimenopause: for example, the two main female hormones, progesterone and estrogen, decline, which affects many other chemical reactions in your body, including the main fat regulator insulin and the neurotransmitter serotonin. Research shows that when women are low in estrogen and progesterone, they are often low in serotonin as well. Progesterone protects brain cells that are involved in the production of serotonin, so progesterone's rapid decline during the perimenopausal years lowers the production of serotonin. While the exact function isn't yet understood, many experts speculate that estrogen helps the cells in your body become more receptive to producing serotonin, which is why many women who are entering the perimenopause years and experiencing this decline in estrogen report that they have cravings for carbs.

Remember, your body is always striving to level out any imbalances. That's why when your progesterone and estrogen decrease, causing lower serotonin levels, you feel down and your brain craves Sugar Calories to elevate your insulin levels, causing your impulse control and willpower to plummet. Your body is trying to restore equilibrium because its alarm bells are going off. Your body doesn't know that uncontrolled sugar binges aren't good; it only knows that by causing you to crave the foods that will increase your insulin, it will get tryptophan so it can make serotonin.

This is key, because with the right knowledge, you can address these biological issues and return your body to equilibrium without gaining weight or having uncontrollable cravings.

The unfair truth is when you compare men and women throughout their lives, women are much more likely to suffer due to disorders related to serotonin deficiencies. But by putting together these two essential ingredients—the Slim and the Happy—it equals long-term weight-loss success.

Now it's time to get started eating the Happy Hormones, Slim Belly™ way.

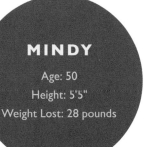

MINDY

Age: 50
Height: 5'5"
Weight Lost: 28 pounds

I'd been on Weight Watchers for some time, but my weight loss had stalled. I always felt like my points went too fast, and I'd be starving before and after dinner, which led to me giving in to sugary and starchy foods. Then I saw Jorge on TV, and his message sounded right up my alley.

BEST STRATEGY:

Prep ahead. I learned that many of the HHSB plan's recipes—such as the lasagna cups, spinach macaroni bites, and rice and bean stuffed peppers—could be doubled or tripled, made ahead of time, and frozen to have on hand for busy days.

BIGGEST CHALLENGE:

I had to change my diet mentality. I was so used to feeling hungry and deprived on other diets that I wasn't sure that this plan could work. Feeling so full and satisfied actually frightened me at first; I thought I must be gaining weight, but at the end of the first week I was 7 pounds lighter. Success!

GREATEST PAYOFF:

My friends and family tell me I look slimmer and happier—and that's exactly how I feel. I know it is because my hormones are in balance, and I really am happy. I still have weight to lose, and I'm confident it will come off easily because I love eating this way.

4

the solution:
Your Carb Cycling Plan

t's time for action. What you'll find in this chapter is an outline for the next several weeks of your life on your journey to optimal health and lasting weight loss. You'll find three plans that are designed to match your different moods, level of impulse control, and cravings, as well as detailed explanations for how to put each plan to use. Weekly shopping lists are included for your convenience, so you can cross one more thing off your to-do list. For those days when your schedule is jam-packed, I've also created two on-the-go menus—one for Slim Days and one for Happy Days (see pages 68 and 69). Finally, I've done all the Sugar Calorie calculations for you, so all you have to do is follow the meal plans as charted below, and watch as you lose up to 7 pounds the first week and 2 pounds weekly!

THE SOLUTION = 2 SLIM DAYS & 5 HAPPY DAYS

My Carb Cycling Plan is the perfect way to get the results you want, without feeling starved, deprived, or depressed. I've named this the Carb Cycling Plan because you strictly limit Sugar Calories (such as carbs) for only two days a week, then you cycle back in the right kind of Sugar Calories, in the right amounts, for the remaining five days of the week. It's so simple—you just alternate between following the Slim Days eating plan for two consecutive days a week, then the Happy Days eating plan for the next five, and the weight just melts away!

CALCULATING SUGAR CALORIES

While I've done all the math for you on the menus in this chapter, it's easy to calculate the amount of Sugar Calories in an item: Simply multiply the total carbohydrate grams on an item's nutritional label by 4. (Sugar grams are already included in an item's total carbohydrate amount, so they don't need to be counted separately.) If the carbohydrate amount has a decimal, round up your answer after multiplying.

carbohydrate grams x 4 = Sugar Calories

The result of cycling these two different styles of eating will be increased energy, elevated feelings of happiness, and rapid weight loss and fat burning—all without the cravings that have set you up to fail in the past. This is the middle path, the one that matches the way your body was meant to work. You'll balance the hormones that caused the negative effects, while increasing the neurotransmitters that keep you feeling your best. By eating the Carb Cycling way, you'll keep your body happy and slim.

WHAT ARE FREEBIE FLOURS?

Foods made with white, whole-wheat, and other grain-based flours contain high levels of carbohydrates that will quickly eat up your daily allotment of Sugar Calories, spike your levels of insulin, and lead to weight gain and belly fat. Fortunately, I've discovered three fantastic, low-carb flours that have zero Sugar Calories and can be used in a variety of foods, such as muffins, cakes, pancakes, chips, crackers, breads, and breading for fried foods. I call them Freebie Flours, and they are available online, at health-food stores, and at many grocery stores. Not only will these Freebie Flours accelerate your weight loss, they are gluten-free and full of nutrients, antioxidants, and fiber.

Get the scoop on these highly nutritious replacements:

- **Coconut flour:** Full of fiber and low in carbohydrates, this flour makes a great replacement breading for fried chicken and other fried foods; it creates a wonderful crust and has a natural nutty sweetness to it. Coconut flour also makes great muffins, cakes, and breads. Coconut has been shown to raise levels of "healthy" cholesterol (HDL).

- **Flax flour:** This powerhouse of nutrients, also called flaxseed meal, contains high levels of natural antioxidants, fiber, and healthy omega-3 fatty acids that have been shown to improve hair growth, promote younger-looking skin, reduce the risk of cancers and diabetes, protect against heart disease, relieve menopausal symptoms, promote healthy bowel movements, and support the immune system. Flaxseed flour makes a great nutty-tasting replacement for flour in pancakes, muffins, and waffles.

- **Almond flour:** Almond flour is made from skinless, blanched, finely ground almonds. This Freebie Flour has a moist texture and rich buttery flavor that makes great cakes and cookies. It can also be used to make crackers and chips. This flour is high in fiber, vitamin E, and magnesium. Magnesium has been shown to improve mood and reduce menopausal symptoms, and vitamin E has been shown to improve heart health.

For recipe ideas using these flours, visit www.jorgecruise.com.

HOW YOUR CARB CYCLING PLAN WORKS

2 SLIM DAYS

On two consecutive days of the week, you will eat delicious meals that are rich in protein, healthy fats, and vegetables. Your meals should be mostly made up of items from the Freebie Foods lists in Chapter 7; the recipes I've included for your Slim Days are constructed in this way. Freebie Foods are healthy proteins, fats, vegetables, and foods made from selected low-carb flours that I call "Freebie Flours"; they are so low in Sugar Calories, and so high in nutrients, that they don't need to be tracked. In other words, Freebie Foods are "free." That said, I'm not giving you carte blanche to eat 20 slices of bacon and 12 eggs in a single sitting. However, because these foods are highly satisfying, you will tend to naturally eat a reasonable portion. Also, since these foods keep insulin levels low, they liberate fat from your fat cells and help you shed weight quickly.

On these two days, keep your daily allotment of Sugar Calories at or below 100. (Anything on the Freebie list, of course, does not need to be counted.) Keeping under 100 Sugar Calories in a day resets your insulin sensitivity, so you reduce the negative effects of carbs and keep your fat-burning engine turned up to its maximum. The Slim Days menus that I've provided for you have 0 Sugar Calories, so you can add up to 100 Sugar Calories of your choice. Please see Chapter 7 for selections.

I suggest that you start out the week (Monday and Tuesday) with your Slim Days, so that you have full clearance for the rest of the week to be social and optimize your serotonin levels. One way I've found to ensure that these two days are enjoyable and effortless is by incorporating foods made from the low-carb flours that I call Freebie Flours. By using these flours, and the recipes that you'll find in this book and on my site www.jorgecruise.com, you'll enjoy breads, muffins, cakes, and more without a single Sugar Calorie. However, this is completely optional.

5 HAPPY DAYS

After your two Slim Days, you can eat up to 500 Sugar Calories a day for five days in a row. These five Happy Days incorporate a sensible, easy-to-follow diet that optimizes the right Sugar Calories (yes, some are better than others) in the right amounts, so you keep your serotonin quota stocked. This in turn helps you feel your best, keeps your motivation high, and eliminates sugar and carb cravings. Remember that the trick is starting your week with Slim Days because it resets your insulin levels; then, 500 Sugar Calories or less are all you will need to feel fully satisfied during the rest of the week.

During your Happy Days you will eat sumptuous meals that include foods from the Freebie Foods list as well as the healthiest foods from the Sugar Calories list, also found in Chapter 7. On these days you will increase your insulin to a healthy level and boost your serotonin to eliminate cravings, overeating, and negative moods. I've designed the menus so that you get those Sugar Calories from the best sources first. When choosing your own options, you can use the following as a guide, in descending order from most to least ideal:

1. Beans and legumes
2. Starchy vegetables
3. Whole grains
4. Fruits
5. Refined carbs (white bread, rolls, buns)
6. Condiments
7. Treats and desserts

TRACKING YOUR PROGRESS

Before you begin stocking your kitchen and preparing yourself for the planners on the following pages, I want you to take a couple of steps so you have an accurate picture of "you" before you begin this program, and a clear understanding of where you want to go—your goals. Taking a few minutes to create a clear picture of your baseline—your current weight and measurements—and knowing how to track yourself on a weekly basis will set you up for success by providing you with visible, measurable changes that will keep your spirits high. When you can see the inches melt off your body and the scale's number getting lower and lower, your motivation will stay revved up.

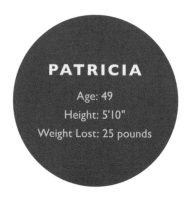

One morning I was watching a bit of news while getting ready for my day, and I saw Jorge on TV talking about a new diet for women over 40. Everything he said hit home for me. Feeling exhausted? Check. Feeling stressed out and sad? Check. Having uncontrollable sugar cravings? Check.

BEST STRATEGY:

Sticking to the plan religiously helped me to not overthink or obsess about food. The menus, shopping lists, and recipes made it so easy.

BIGGEST CHALLENGE:

Lack of regularity. At first I noticed that I was a bit constipated on this food plan, but that was easily remedied. Jorge suggested that I add a couple tablespoons of ground flaxseed to my Nutty Cottage Cheese or to my Jay Robb protein shakes*. I aim to have one of these each day, and now I have no more issues.

GREATEST PAYOFF:

I love how much more energy I have these days. Now I take a Pilates class after my workday, and I love it. I also feel "cleaner" on the inside from ridding myself of all the unnecessary Sugar Calories.

*Note from Jorge: You'll see me recommend Jay Robb protein shakes in later chapters. I love Jay Robb products because they are one of the few healthy, fully sugar-free protein powders on the market. Plus, they are widely available in health-food stores, and online at www.jayrobb.com.

A Word about the Scale

The key to seeing progressive weight loss each week is consistency. I know it is tempting to step on the scale every time you walk past it, but this strategy may backfire because weight can fluctuate on an hourly basis depending on what you eat, what time of the month it is, or how much water you are retaining at a given moment. Sometimes you can weigh 4 pounds or more at night than you did that same morning, but that doesn't reflect your true weight. With that in mind, I believe it is best to weigh yourself under the same circumstances: once a week, first thing in the morning. That way you'll see a truer reflection of the weight you are losing.

Your body mass index (BMI) is a good guide to what your healthy weight should be. It is an estimate of what your body fat is, taking your height and weight into account. (However, it does have its limitations; for example, it doesn't account for a muscular build, so a very fit person can have a high BMI without actually having a high body-fat percentage.) To see what your BMI is and what it should be, use the handy calculator here: www.nhlbi.nih.gov/guidelines/obesity/BMI/bmicalc.htm.

Measuring Your Waist

Grab a fabric or flexible tape measure (available at any drugstore) and suck in your belly as much as you can. Now place the tape measure at belly-button level and measure your waist. According to research, risk of cardiovascular health issues increase when a woman's waist circumference is more than 35 inches (for a man, it's at more than 40 inches). Mark the number, along with your goal number, below, next to the marking for your waist. Also note your current weight and your goal weight below.

It is important to keep an accurate measurement of your waist and weight. When you measure again next week, repeat the same process. No more assessing yourself by eye in the mirror, guessing whether you were sucking it in last week as opposed to this week.

My baseline weight _____   My baseline waist _____

My goal weight _____   My goal waist _____

Now, each week, repeat these actions with your scale and tape measure, and track your progress below:

WEEK 1:   Weight _____   Waist _____

WEEK 2:   Weight _____   Waist _____

WEEK 3:   Weight _____   Waist _____

WEEK 4:   Weight _____   Waist _____

WEEK 5:   Weight _____   Waist _____

WEEK 6:   Weight _____   Waist _____

WEEK 7:   Weight _____   Waist _____

WEEK 8:   Weight _____   Waist _____

WEEK 9:   Weight _____   Waist _____

WEEK 10:   Weight _____   Waist _____

WEEK 11:   Weight _____   Waist _____

WEEK 12:   Weight _____   Waist _____

HAPPY HORMONES, SLIM BELLY™ ONLINE

TOOLS FOR A SLIM BELLY. ALL ONLINE.

Learn how to follow the Happy Hormones, Slim Belly™ program
step-by-step, and get every tool you need
to be successful—all online.

IT GOES WHERE YOU GO.

Whether you're busy with your family or at your job,
you can always access information about
Happy Hormones, Slim Belly™
on your computer or mobile device.

YOU'VE GOT OPTIONS.

You'll get a weekly menu and meal planner as well as
a library of thousands of food lists and recipes.
You'll continue eating what you love—in a healthy way.

Visit HappyHormonesSlimBelly.com to get started online.

HAPPY HORMONES, SLIM BELLY™ WEEK 1

Here we go. This week I want you to just focus on the details of the plan, getting the right ingredients, and being good to yourself. For many women the first week is the easiest because motivation is high, so it's a great time to write down how you are feeling and take notes on what you like about the program, what modifications you made that worked for you, and your progress.

Often, women ignore the inches that they lose on my programs, but these inches reflect fat coming off your body. Since lean muscle weighs more than fat, you may see inches lost, and more room in your jeans, before you see the scale move. Don't discount this! Waist circumference is an important marker for heart health, so remember to measure your waist, and let's get moving.

The weekend before you start the program, set aside some time to clean out your cupboards and fridge, review the shopping lists for each planner below, then hit the store. If you have trigger foods, especially foods high in Sugar Calories (such as cookies, ice cream, chips, white bread, or candy), get a bag and store them out of reach or simply toss them. Making your home a zero-tolerance zone for sugars and refined carbs is a great way to help you stick to your plan.

> **N O T E :** Many items you'll purchase will be used week after week, so feel free to buy more rather than less. For these lists, I've usually put how much of something you'll need for the week, which doesn't always match the sizes that items are sold in. (For example, I write that you'll need 2 tablespoons of cream cheese, but when you go to the store, you'll have to purchase a full container.) Simply purchase the general sizes that the products come in when you stock up on Week 1. Then, for Week 2 and beyond, be sure to inventory your fridge and pantry, and compare them against the lists before going shopping, so you don't end up with too much or too little of something.
>
> Also, while I've calculated the Sugar Calories for you in each of the following menus, remember that brands vary in their ingredients; always be mindful of nutrition labels.

	1 **SLIM**	**2** **SLIM**	**3** **HAPPY**
BREAK-FAST	Breakfast Lasagna & coffee with half-and-half (see page 109) 0 Sugar Calories	Breakfast Shake & coffee with half-and-half (see page 112) 0 Sugar Calories	Ham and Egg Crepe Square & coffee with half-and-half (see page 143) 48 Sugar Calories
SNACK	10 almonds 0 Sugar Calories	¼ cup pumpkin seeds 0 Sugar Calories	10 almonds 0 Sugar Calories
LUNCH	Chicken Salad–Stuffed Tomatoes (see page 121) 0 Sugar Calories	Tuna Cups (see page 124) 0 Sugar Calories	BLT Egg Sandwich (see page 169) 160 Sugar Calories
SNACK	1 string-cheese stick 0 Sugar Calories	1 hard-boiled egg 0 Sugar Calories	1 string-cheese stick 0 Sugar Calories
DINNER	Italian Salad (see page 125) 0 Sugar Calories	Eggplant Rollups (see page 123) 0 Sugar Calories	Spicy Corn Cakes (see page 173) 87 Sugar Calories
TREAT	Sweet Skinny Waffle (see page 217) 0 Sugar Calories	Sweet Skinny Waffle (see page 217) 0 Sugar Calories	Sweet Skinny Waffle (see page 217) 0 Sugar Calories
TOTAL	0 Sugar Calories	0 Sugar Calories	295 Sugar Calories

4 HAPPY	5 HAPPY	6 HAPPY	7 HAPPY
Peanut Butter and Strawberry Toasts & coffee with half-and-half (see page 145) 144 Sugar Calories	Baja Toast & coffee with half-and-half (see page 147) 126 Sugar Calories	Ham and Egg Crepe Square & coffee with half-and-half (see page 143) 48 Sugar Calories	Tasty Toast & coffee with half-and-half (see page 146) 127 Sugar Calories
¼ cup pumpkin seeds 0 Sugar Calories	10 almonds 0 Sugar Calories	¼ cup pumpkin seeds 0 Sugar Calories	10 almonds 0 Sugar Calories
Sweet Spinach Salad (see page 171) 139 Sugar Calories	Open-Faced Avocado Sandwich (see page 167) 65 Sugar Calories	Feta Pita Pizza (see page 170) 67 Sugar Calories	Sweet Spinach Salad (see page 171) 139 Sugar Calories
1 hard-boiled egg 0 Sugar Calories	1 string-cheese stick 0 Sugar Calories	1 hard-boiled egg 0 Sugar Calories	1 string-cheese stick 0 Sugar Calories
Zucchini Linguine (see page 176) 164 Sugar Calories	Lasagna Cups (see page 175) 119 Sugar Calories	Catch of the Day (see page 177) 35 Sugar Calories	Zucchini Linguine (see page 176) 164 Sugar Calories
Sweet Skinny Waffle (see page 217) 0 Sugar Calories	Sweet Skinny Waffle (see page 217) 0 Sugar Calories	Sweet Skinny Waffle (see page 217) 0 Sugar Calories	Sweet Skinny Waffle (see page 217) 0 Sugar Calories
447 Sugar Calories	310 Sugar Calories	150 Sugar Calories	430 Sugar Calories

carb cycling shopping list

PRODUCE

16-oz. package of
  baby spinach

2 heads of romaine

2 avocados

I yellow zucchini

2 medium zucchinis

I package mushrooms

I small package of
  cherry tomatoes

2 tomatoes

I ear corn

I head broccoli

I large eggplant

3 radishes

I small carton of
  strawberries

2 lemons

I lime

I pear

I apple

I large onion

I small red onion

I head of garlic

scallions

fresh basil

fresh parsley

fresh cilantro

MEAT/FISH

12 eggs

4 oz. breakfast
  sausage

4 strips bacon

chicken, precooked or
  rotisserie (at least
  1½ cups worth)

I can tuna

4 slices pepperoni

2 slices ham

I oz. ground beef

I halibut fillet

DAIRY

I pint half-and-half

4 string-cheese sticks

½ pint whipping cream

¾ cup ricotta cheese

16 oz. Parmesan,
  grated

16 oz. mozzarella,
  shredded

½ cup goat cheese

1 tsp. buttermilk

1 carton feta cheese, crumbles

1 container whipped cream

2 Tbsp. cream cheese

½ cup blue cheese, crumbles

1 slice pepper Jack cheese

1 slice provolone

1 package of butter

OTHER

1 pint unsweetened coconut milk

1 small baguette

1 loaf whole-grain bread

1 loaf pumpernickel bread

1 loaf whole-wheat bread

1 loaf whole-wheat pita bread

1 package small artisan rolls

1 oz. chopped pecans

2 oz. almonds

4 oz. pumpkin seeds

1 jar or container of black or Greek olives, pitted and sliced

1 jar sun-dried tomatoes, packed in oil

1 jar Alfredo sauce

1 jar marinara sauce, no sugar added

1 jar sugar-free fruit spread

1 jar peanut butter

16-oz. package linguine

1 package wonton wrappers

1 bag Strawberry Jay Robb whey protein

wild rice

cornmeal

all-purpose flour

almond flour

olive oil

canola oil

coffee

mayonnaise

garlic powder

onion powder

cumin

chili powder

salt

pepper

dried oregano

dried basil

baking powder

baking soda

Truvia packets

stevia powder

Barlean's The Essential Woman Chocolate Mint Swirl

7 Skinny Waffles™ (skinnywaffle.com)

QUICK TIP

Choose breads with no more than 15 grams of carbs (60 Sugar Calories) per serving.

HAPPY HORMONES, SLIM BELLY™ WEEK 2

So, how did it go? Did you write down the weight and inches you lost? Many of you will have seen a big change in the scale by this point, but don't get discouraged if it was smaller than you'd like. Your body is unique, and the way it responds will be different for each beautiful one of you. My experience is that those who would like to lose a lot of weight, especially those who used to drink lots of sugary beverages and sodas, will see a big change. If you are only trying to lose a small amount of weight, you may lose less, but you *will* still lose the weight, so don't stop.

If you'd like to see more weight loss but aren't ready to dive into the Extra-Slim Planner, you can leave out a few of the bread servings on your Happy Days. I only want you to do this when you feel up to it, but the fewer Sugar Calories you have, the less fat your body will hang on to. On the other hand, if the weight is coming off just fine but you are feeling a bit low, make sure you're getting all of your carb servings. Additionally, as we just discussed, you may want to space out your carbs to get an extra boost in your happy hormones.

Remember, before doing your grocery shopping for Week 2, take time to scan your cupboards and refrigerator. You may now have some of the staples that you'll find on the following shopping list. And you'll be able to make a list of what you need. Also, see the box in this chapter titled "Quick Tips for Staying on Track" for ideas on how to plan ahead and keep yourself on track all week long. Make sure to review the recipes—are there any that you can make in advance and freeze? If so, and you have time on Sunday, plan on making a few recipes so you can save time when the week gets jammed up.

WEEK 2: CARB CYCLING MEAL PLANNER

	1 SLIM	2 SLIM	3 HAPPY
BREAK-FAST	Traditional Skinny Waffle & coffee with half-and-half (see page 111) 0 Sugar Calories	Breakfast Shake & coffee with half-and-half (see page 112) 0 Sugar Calories	Maple Bacon Sandwich & coffee with half-and-half (see page 149) 80 Sugar Calories
SNACK	3 celery sticks spread with cream cheese 0 Sugar Calories	10 macadamia nuts 0 Sugar Calories	3 celery sticks spread with cream cheese 0 Sugar Calories
LUNCH	Classic Wedge Salad (see page 127) 0 Sugar Calories	Italian Salad (see page 125) 0 Sugar Calories	Heirloom Tomato Toasts (see page 179) 160 Sugar Calories
SNACK	1 string-cheese stick 0 Sugar Calories	1 slice deli turkey & 1 slice cheddar 0 Sugar Calories	1 string-cheese stick 0 Sugar Calories
DINNER	Basil Pesto Pizza (see page 129) 0 Sugar Calories	Turkey Caesar Salad (see page 130) 0 Sugar Calories	Sweet Potato Skins (see page 185) 79 Sugar Calories
TREAT	2-Minute Cake (see page 215) 0 Sugar Calories	2-Minute Cake (see page 215) 0 Sugar Calories	2-Minute Cake (see page 215) 0 Sugar Calories
TOTAL	0 Sugar Calories	0 Sugar Calories	319 Sugar Calories

4 HAPPY	5 HAPPY	6 HAPPY	7 HAPPY
Chicks on a Nest & coffee with half-and-half (see page 152) 120 Sugar Calories	Sunshine Wrap & coffee with half-and-half (see page 151) 42 Sugar Calories	Kale and Goat Cheese Scramble & coffee with half-and-half (see page 153) 60 Sugar Calories	Maple Bacon Sandwich & coffee with half-and-half (see page 149) 80 Sugar Calories
10 macadamia nuts 0 Sugar Calories	3 celery sticks spread with cream cheese 0 Sugar Calories	10 macadamia nuts 0 Sugar Calories	3 celery sticks spread with cream cheese 0 Sugar Calories
Rockin' Ravioli (see page 182) 100 Sugar Calories	Rice and Bean Stuffed Pepper (see page 181) 120 Sugar Calories	Prosciutto Wrap (see page 183) 80 Sugar Calories	Heirloom Tomato Toasts (see page 179) 160 Sugar Calories
1 slice deli turkey & 1 slice cheddar 0 Sugar Calories	1 string-cheese stick 0 Sugar Calories	1 slice deli turkey & 1 slice cheddar 0 Sugar Calories	1 string-cheese stick 0 Sugar Calories
Penne Marinara (see page 188) 156 Sugar Calories	Sautéed Scallops (see page 187) 72 Sugar Calories	Savory Kebab (see page 189) 90 Sugar Calories	Sweet Potato Skins (see page 185) 79 Sugar Calories
2-Minute Cake (see page 215) 0 Sugar Calories	2-Minute Cake (see page 215) 0 Sugar Calories	2-Minute Cake (see page 215) 0 Sugar Calories	2-Minute Cake (see page 215) 0 Sugar Calories
376 Sugar Calories	234 Sugar Calories	230 Sugar Calories	319 Sugar Calories

carb cycling shopping list

PRODUCE

½ head iceberg lettuce

1 cup kale

3 cups romaine, shredded

3¾ cups spinach

¼ cup arugula

¼ cup alfalfa sprouts

5 cherry tomatoes

2 tomatoes (or 1 tomato and 4 heirloom tomatoes)

½ head cauliflower

½ cup eggplant

3 asparagus stalks

1 sweet potato

1 potato

1 celery stalk

2 red bell peppers

1 head broccoli

1 onion

2 Tbsp. red onion, chopped

4 garlic cloves

1 shallot

1 Tbsp. chives

¼ cup fresh basil, chopped

MEAT/FISH

17 eggs

8 strips bacon (you can make 6 of these strips maple bacon)

1 cup chicken, sliced

3 oz. chicken breast

4 slices pepperoni

1 Italian sausage

¼ cup deli turkey, shredded

3 slices prosciutto

3–6 scallops

DAIRY

4 string-cheese sticks

¼ cup cheddar cheese, grated

4 slices cheddar

2 Tbsp. pepper Jack cheese, shredded

2 Tbsp. blue cheese, crumbles

1¼ cups mozzarella

¾ cup goat cheese

½ cup feta cheese

2 Tbsp. cream cheese

2 Tbsp. sour cream

Parmesan cheese

half-and-half

butter

whipping cream

OTHER

1 small whole-grain baguette

3 slices whole-grain bread

1 package small artisan rolls

1 whole-wheat wrap

1 spinach tortilla wrap

5 whole-wheat cheese ravioli

2 oz. whole-wheat penne pasta

¾ cup brown rice

¼ cup black beans

¼ cup chickpeas

40 almonds

¾ cup pumpkin seeds

2 Tbsp. pine nuts

2 Tbsp. blue cheese dressing, no sugar added

2 Tbsp. Caesar dressing

¼ cup marinara sauce, no sugar added

⅓ cup pesto

2 Tbsp. soy sauce

½ tsp. garlic salt

1 tsp. cumin

1 cup almond flour

½ cup unsweetened cocoa powder

½ cup Truvia Baking Blend

2 packets Truvia

unsweetened almond milk

coffee

Jay Robb vanilla whey protein

baking powder

baking soda

coconut oil

dried oregano

dried basil

olive oil

salt

pepper

1 Skinny Waffle™ (skinnywaffle.com)

Skinny Maple Syrup™ (skinnymaplesyrup .com)

GET A NATURAL HIGH

Tricks and Tips for Feeling Your Best
with non-food strategies for spiking serotonin

— Get enough light every day: Natural sunlight and light-therapy lamps help keep serotonin levels maximized. Aim to get outside for a 30-minute walk, some gardening or yard work, or at least a seat in the sun. Don't put on sunscreen for these 30 minutes because it blocks the health effects of sunshine; however, if you will be out for a prolonged period of time, do lather up.

— Move: In Chapter 8, I discuss how exercise can boost your serotonin levels and increase your energy. This doesn't mean running marathons or becoming a bodybuilder; simply including approximately 20 minutes of walking three times a week can help you stay on track with your weight-loss goals. In addition, in Chapter 8 I've included a simple strength-training routine because research does show that building even a small amount of muscle can increase your energy, make you look slimmer, and increase serotonin.

— Sleep: Your serotonin levels and the amount of sleep you get are intimately related. If you are sleep deprived (and, according to research, the majority of adults are), then chances are that you may be short on serotonin as well. Lack of sleep lowers your ability to control impulses, and increases your cravings for highly refined carbs and sugars. To make sure you feel your best, it is always smart to keep your bedroom reserved for only two activities: sleep and sex. Also, make sure your bedroom is as dark as possible, because even a small amount of light can stimulate your brain to produce hormones that wake you up or keep you from relaxing. Cover any digital clocks or computer screens, and never watch TV in bed; otherwise, your brain will associate sleep time with TV time—and, bingo, you're up all night.

Yahoo! You're doing so great. Week 3 can be a challenge because the newness of the program is wearing off and you may be losing a bit of motivation. So it's time to ramp up your inspiration and enthusiasm.

Try the following: Take out a piece of paper and a pen and set a timer for five minutes. Divide the paper into three columns, and at the top write *Mental, Physical,* and *Emotional.* Now start writing all the reasons you want to lose weight. Under *Mental* you might write things such as "clarity of mind, better memory, ability to focus, positive thinking." Under *Physical* the words might be "lower blood pressure, have more energy to exercise, be able to play with my grandkids," and under *Emotional* you might write "increased serenity, decreased mood swings, more relaxed." Save this list or post it on your fridge or bathroom mirror as an inspiring reminder of all the things you gain from the program in addition to losing weight.

The weekend before Week 3, scan your kitchen supplies and make a list of what you need from the following shopping list. Think about how you are feeling about particular foods and drinks. Have you been craving soda? If so, pick up some sparkling water and lemons so you can "feed" your desire for a bubbly beverage without the sugar or chemicals. Have you been having sugar cravings? Be sure to have berries on hand as a snack on Happy Days. The longer you're away from refined sugars, the sweeter natural foods will taste to you. If you have time, precook some chicken breasts or other meats in the upcoming recipes to save you time when your schedule gets packed.

	1 SLIM	2 SLIM	3 HAPPY
BREAK-FAST	Sautéed Vegetable Frittata & coffee with half-and-half (see page 115) 0 Sugar Calories	Cinnamon-Nut Cottage Cheese & coffee with half-and-half (see page 118) 0 Sugar Calories	Bacon Eggs Benedict & coffee with half-and-half (see page 155) 50 Sugar Calories
SNACK	10 almonds 0 Sugar Calories	¼ cup sunflower seeds 0 Sugar Calories	10 almonds 0 Sugar Calories
LUNCH	Chicken Caprese Stacks (see page 133) 0 Sugar Calories	Dijon Salmon (see page 131) 0 Sugar Calories	Steak and Goat Cheese Quesadilla (see page 191) 127 Sugar Calories
SNACK	1 string-cheese stick 0 Sugar Calories	1 hard-boiled egg 0 Sugar Calories	1 string-cheese stick 0 Sugar Calories
DINNER	Zucchini Boats (see page 135) 0 Sugar Calories	Steak Kebab (see page 136) 0 Sugar Calories	Sweet Kale Wrap (see page 193) 184 Sugar Calories
TREAT	Sweet Skinny Waffle (see page 217) 0 Sugar Calories	Sweet Skinny Waffle (see page 217) 0 Sugar Calories	Sweet Skinny Waffle (see page 217) 0 Sugar Calories
TOTAL	0 Sugar Calories	0 Sugar Calories	361 Sugar Calories

4 HAPPY	5 HAPPY	6 HAPPY	7 HAPPY
Ricotta Omelet & coffee with half-and-half (see page 158)	Nutty Oatmeal & coffee with half-and-half (see page 157)	Fruity Yogurt & coffee with half-and-half (see page 159)	Bacon Eggs Benedict & coffee with half-and-half (see page 155)
104 Sugar Calories	120 Sugar Calories	33 Sugar Calories	50 Sugar Calories
¼ cup sunflower seeds	10 almonds	¼ cup sunflower seeds	10 almonds
0 Sugar Calories	0 Sugar Calories	0 Sugar Calories	0 Sugar Calories
Feta Turkey Burger (see page 194)	Spinach Pasta with Shrimp (see page 197)	Chicken Spanish Wrap (see page 200)	Steak and Goat Cheese Quesadilla (see page 191)
120 Sugar Calories	53 Sugar Calories	80 Sugar Calories	127 Sugar Calories
1 hard-boiled egg	1 string-cheese stick	1 hard-boiled egg	1 string-cheese stick
0 Sugar Calories	0 Sugar Calories	0 Sugar Calories	0 Sugar Calories
Citrus Shrimp (see page 195)	Italian Chicken Pita (see page 201)	Bacon Spaghetti with Garlic Croutons (see page 199)	Sweet Kale Wrap (see page 193)
90 Sugar Calories	150 Sugar Calories	168 Sugar Calories	184 Sugar Calories
Sweet Skinny Waffle (see page 217)	Sweet Skinny Waffle (see page 217)	Sweet Skinny Waffle (see page 217)	Sweet Skinny Waffle (see page 217)
0 Sugar Calories	0 Sugar Calories	0 Sugar Calories	0 Sugar Calories
314 Sugar Calories	323 Sugar Calories	281 Sugar Calories	361 Sugar Calories

carb cycling shopping list

PRODUCE

¼ cup arugula	10 cherry tomatoes	1 lime
3 cups spinach	2 tsp. jalapeños	1 Tbsp. blackberries
½ cup mixed greens	½ cup kale	1 Tbsp. blueberries
shredded lettuce	½ cup mushrooms	1 mango
4 asparagus stalks	1 onion	1 garlic clove
1 avocado	1 red onion	fresh basil
1 red bell pepper	1 zucchini	fresh cilantro
1 tomato	1 lemon	fresh parsley

MEAT/FISH

15 eggs	1 turkey patty	2½ chicken breasts
1 salmon fillet	3 oz. steak	8 slices bacon
9 medium shrimp	6 strips flank steak	

DAIRY

½ cup cottage cheese	4 string-cheese sticks	1 Tbsp. sour cream
3 Tbsp. cheddar cheese	2 Tbsp. feta cheese	half-and-half
	¼ cup goat cheese	butter
1 slice mozzarella	2 Tbsp. ricotta cheese	whipping cream
2 slices provolone	¼ cup Greek yogurt	

OTHER

unsweetened vanilla almond milk

1 whole-wheat pita

1 whole-wheat hamburger bun

2 English muffins

5 garlic croutons

7 whole-wheat tortillas

¾ cup whole-wheat spaghetti

¾ cup spinach pasta

½ cup brown rice

¼ cup steel-cut oats

1 can black beans

40 almonds

2 Tbsp. pecans

¾ cup sunflower seeds

1 Tbsp. walnuts

2 Tbsp. unsweetened coconut flakes

1 Tbsp. Dijon mustard

1 Tbsp. mayonnaise

1 Tbsp. marinara sauce, no sugar added

hummus

Truvia

stevia powder

salt

pepper

olive oil

nonstick cooking spray

cinnamon

curry powder

red pepper flakes

dried thyme

red wine vinegar

balsamic vinegar

coffee

7 Skinny Waffles™ (skinnywaffle.com)

Barlean's The Essential Woman Chocolate Mint Swirl

HAPPY HORMONES, SLIM BELLY WEEK 4

Congratulations! You've been working hard at getting slim and staying happy. This week is a great week to add some fitness into your routine.

Please see Chapter 8 for the best way to incorporate movement to feel your best and help you stay on track toward your goals. Just remember that exercise must feel good and be something you enjoy doing—otherwise it will backfire. That said, even if you've always hated exercise, don't think that what I have to say in Chapter 8 isn't for you. This isn't about hourlong workout sessions, or lifting weights that would make Arnold gag—this is about finding ways to make exercise fun and doable, and I've got tons of great tips for you.

The weekend before Week 4, read Chapter 8, and mark on your calendar at least three times when you will get out and walk or try the strength-training exercises. Plan your shopping lists, and prepackage snacks for a successful week. I'd also suggest reviewing Chapter 5, which discusses how you'll continue to successfully lose weight with the Happy Hormones, Slim Belly™ plan so you will be prepped for the coming weeks and months.

WEEK 4: CARB CYCLING MEAL PLANNER

	1 SLIM	2 SLIM	3 HAPPY
BREAK-FAST	Poached Prosciutto & coffee with half-and-half (see page 117) 0 Sugar Calories	Nutty Cottage Cheese & coffee with half-and-half (see page 119) 0 Sugar Calories	Egg-in-a-Hole Sandwich & coffee with half-and-half (see page 161) 53 Sugar Calories
SNACK	3 celery sticks dipped in mustard 0 Sugar Calories	10 pecans 0 Sugar Calories	3 celery sticks dipped in mustard 0 Sugar Calories
LUNCH	Jalapeño Bites (see page 139) 0 Sugar Calories	Green Greek Salad (see page 137) 0 Sugar Calories	Spinach Macaroni Bites (see page 203) 148 Sugar Calories
SNACK	10 macadamia nuts 0 Sugar Calories	1 slice deli turkey & 1 slice cheddar cheese 0 Sugar Calories	10 macadamia nuts 0 Sugar Calories
DINNER	Stuffed Salmon (see page 141) 0 Sugar Calories	Tuna Cups (see page 124) 0 Sugar Calories	Spinach Bacon Quesadilla (see page 209) 82 Sugar Calories
TREAT	2-Minute Cake (see page 215) 0 Sugar Calories	2-Minute Cake (see page 215) 0 Sugar Calories	2-Minute Cake (see page 215) 0 Sugar Calories
TOTAL	0 Sugar Calories	0 Sugar Calories	283 Sugar Calories

4 HAPPY	5 HAPPY	6 HAPPY	7 HAPPY
Fruit and Nut Yogurt & coffee with half-and-half (see page 164) 8 Sugar Calories	Baked Oatmeal Muffins & coffee with half-and-half (see page 163) 78 Sugar Calories	Ricotta Toast & coffee with half-and-half (see page 165) 102 Sugar Calories	Egg-in-a-Hole Sandwich & coffee with half-and-half (see page 161) 53 Sugar Calories
10 pecans 0 Sugar Calories	3 celery sticks dipped in mustard 0 Sugar Calories	10 pecans 0 Sugar Calories	3 celery sticks dipped in mustard 0 Sugar Calories
Chicken Stir-fry (see page 206) 99 Sugar Calories	Guacamole Grilled Cheese (see page 205) 120 Sugar Calories	Pig in a Wrap (see page 207) 86 Sugar Calories	Spinach Macaroni Bites (see page 203) 148 Sugar Calories
1 slice deli turkey & 1 slice cheddar cheese 0 Sugar Calories	10 macadamia nuts 0 Sugar Calories	1 slice deli turkey & 1 slice cheddar cheese 0 Sugar Calories	10 macadamia nuts 0 Sugar Calories
Pesto Pita Pizza (see page 212) 70 Sugar Calories	Mediterranean Tacos (see page 211) 54 Sugar Calories	Tuna Melt (see page 213) 60 Sugar Calories	Spinach Bacon Quesadilla (see page 209) 82 Sugar Calories
2-Minute Cake (see page 215) 0 Sugar Calories	2-Minute Cake (see page 215) 0 Sugar Calories	2-Minute Cake (see page 215) 0 Sugar Calories	2-Minute Cake (see page 215) 0 Sugar Calories
177 Sugar Calories	252 Sugar Calories	198 Sugar Calories	283 Sugar Calories

WEEK 4

carb cycling shopping list

PRODUCE

2 cups arugula

2 romaine lettuce
leaves

½ cup shredded
romaine

3½ cups spinach

2 avocados

¼ cup broccoli

¼ carrot

1 bunch celery

½ cucumber

2 jalapeño peppers

3 Tbsp. onion,
chopped

2 Tbsp. red onion,
chopped

2 tomatoes

5 cherry tomatoes

1 lemon

lime juice

3 strawberries

1 banana

1 cup blueberries

½ Tbsp. ginger

2 garlic cloves

fresh cilantro

fresh dill

fresh basil

MEAT/FISH

9 eggs

1 mahi mahi fillet

1 salmon fillet (3–4 oz.)

10 strips bacon

2 slices Canadian
bacon

3 chicken breasts

3 slices deli turkey

4 slices prosciutto

1½ cans tuna

DAIRY

¼ cup ricotta cheese

¼ cup feta cheese

1 Tbsp. creamy goat
cheese

cheddar cheese
(9 slices and 2 Tbsp.
shredded)

½ cup cottage cheese

¼ cup cream cheese

¼ cup plain Greek
yogurt

mozzarella cheese

Parmesan cheese

butter

half-and-half

whipping cream

OTHER

5 slices whole-grain
bread

1 whole-wheat English
muffin

½ whole-wheat pita

3 whole-wheat torti-
llas (wraps)

2 small corn tortillas

2 cups whole-wheat
macaroni noodles

¼ cup quinoa

½ cup rice

16 oz. old-fashioned
oats

¼ cup almonds

40 macadamia nuts

30 pecans

1⅓ cup unsweetened
applesauce

1 Tbsp. black olives

5 Kalamata olives,
pitted

1 tsp. pesto

2 Tbsp. pico de gallo

1 Tbsp. salsa

2 Tbsp. sugar-free
fruit preserves

1 tsp. vanilla extract

¼ cup ground
flaxseed

½ cup unsweetened
cocoa powder

4 packets stevia

3 packets Truvia

½ cup Truvia Baking
Blend

almond flour

baking powder

baking soda

coconut oil

olive oil

salt

pepper

coffee

oregano

cinnamon

mayonnaise

mustard

white vinegar

red wine vinegar

nonstick cooking
spray

4 toothpicks

ON-THE-GO EATING

For days when you don't have time to cook, choose one of the following menu plans—Happy or Slim—depending on which cycle you are following.

HAPPY DAYS ON-THE-GO

Just because it's a "happy day" doesn't mean it isn't busy, so here are options you can choose that keep you at a healthy carb level even when you're on the run from dawn till dusk. You can use these ideas in place of any of the Happy food-plan days—or, if your whole day isn't busy, you can just swap out one meal for another. These meals are simple and can be ordered at most restaurants, as well as easily prepared at home to take with you for a busy day.

HAPPY ON-THE-GO MENU

Breakfast
3 eggs, any style
2 pieces of toast with butter
(Consider boiling some eggs the night before, so you can take them with you.)

Snack
Small handful of walnuts, almonds, or peanuts

Lunch
Tuna or chicken salad on one pita bread, or open-faced on a slice of bread, with lettuce and tomato
(You can also order a salad and have this on the side.)

Snack
1 cup cottage cheese

Dinner
Sautéed chicken, fish, or steak; with ½ cup brown rice, and broccoli
(or another low-sugar vegetable such as asparagus or spinach)

Treat
85% cacao or higher dark chocolate

SLIM DAYS ON-THE-GO

Here are Slim Day menu options for those jam-packed days when you just don't have time to cook. This menu can be used in place of any of the Slim menu days. All these meals can be simply prepared at home or ordered at most restaurants. If you are eating out and feeling tempted, I suggest not even looking at a menu—just make your request, and most establishments will be happy to help.

SLIM ON-THE-GO MENU

Breakfast
2 eggs, any style,
with avocado and mushrooms
(or sautéed veggies of your choice)

Snack
1 piece string cheese

Lunch
Lettuce-wrapped hamburger patty with
avocado and cucumbers

Snack
10 almonds or a small handful of
dry-roasted peanuts

Dinner
Grilled chicken, steak, or fish;
with a side of low-sugar vegetables,
with butter

Treat
85% cacao or higher dark chocolate

A CUSTOMIZED PLAN FOR YOU

While the core of Happy Hormones, Slim Belly™ is the Carb Cycling Plan, I've also included two variations that address some of the hormonal fluctuations and resulting moods that women over 40 experience. The end goal of this program is sustainable weight loss—and that calls for a plan for any mood that may arise. Below are the breakdowns for each variation of the Carb Cycling Plan, and detailed menus and shopping lists for your next month of eating.

— **THE EXTRA-HAPPY PLAN:** This eating strategy is designed for those weeks when life seems overwhelming, and you feel like you might just dive into the first pint of Ben & Jerry's ice cream that crosses your path. (See box: "When Should I Choose the Extra-Happy Meal Plan?" on the next page.) On this plan you'll get to eat up to 500 Sugar Calories a day for all seven days of the week, and you will still see weight loss—it will just be more moderate than on the recommended Carb Cycling Plan. This plan follows the design of my successful Belly Fat Cure™ books. Remember that moderate weight loss is great, especially on a week when you are feeling at high risk for emotional eating or sugar bingeing.

— **THE EXTRA-SLIM PLAN:** Here you'll eat 100 Sugar Calories a day, every day of the week. This plan is modeled after my diet The 100™ and is designed for maximum weight loss, but I want you to use this only on weeks when you are feeling supermotivated and having no sugar cravings. Check in with yourself: if you can pass on the roll with your salad with no problem, then the Extra-Slim Plan may work for you this week.

When Should I Choose the Extra-Happy Meal Plan?

This is the plan to choose when life feels overwhelming. This is the plan for you if you're under 40 and experiencing PMS (often the week before you begin your period), or if you're running into these physical, emotional, or behavioral issues:

- Trouble sleeping

- Muscle tension or aches

- Migraines or headaches

- Gastrointestinal disturbances, including nervous stomach, irritable bowel syndrome (IBS) symptoms, or diarrhea

- Excessive fatigue or exhaustion

- Excessive anxiety or worry

- Loss of enthusiasm in the Carb Cycling program

- Feeling sad or blue

- Feeling overly irritable

- Difficulty sticking to exercise goals

- Extreme carb or sugar cravings

For days when you are feeling really down, some Sugar Calories at certain times of the day will give your serotonin (your happy-hormone booster) an extra kick. The tricky thing is that you need to eat protein to get the amino acid tryptophan, which is the precursor of serotonin. Interestingly, the actual serotonin boost comes from Sugar Calories—and this effect is enhanced when you separate your protein from your carbs.

Based on research, the best way to make this work for you is to eat protein and fats to get lots of tryptophan in your body, wait three hours, and then eat a healthy Sugar Calorie–based snack, which ushers the tryptophan into your brain where it can boost your serotonin levels. This also works when you eat protein with dinner, then start your day with a breakfast of carbs only.

Here's an example of how you'd do it.

- *Breakfast (serotonin-boosting Sugar Calories):* Two slices of toast topped with sliced strawberries or a half of a banana.

- *Snack (protein):* Three hours after your first meal, have one piece of string cheese; a boiled egg; or a small handful of walnuts, almonds, or peanuts.

- *Lunch (Sugar Calories and protein):* Choose a lunch from any day on the Extra-Happy Menu.

- *Snack (serotonin-boosting Sugar Calories):* Three hours after lunch, have a piece of whole-grain toast with half a banana mashed on top.

- *Dinner (carbs and protein):* Three hours after your snack, choose a dinner from any day on the Extra-Happy Menu.

- *Treat:* One glass of wine (5 oz.) and/or a piece of Two-Minute Cake.

You can repeat this style of eating for as many days as you like while using the Extra-Happy Menu or on the Happy Days from the Carb Cycling Menu.

	1 HAPPY	2 HAPPY	3 HAPPY
BREAK-FAST	Ham and Egg Crepe Square & coffee with half-and-half (see page 143) 48 Sugar Calories	Peanut Butter and Strawberry Toasts & coffee with half-and-half (see page 145) 144 Sugar Calories	Baja Toast & coffee with half-and-half (see page 147) 126 Sugar Calories
SNACK	10 almonds 0 Sugar Calories	¼ cup pumpkin seeds 0 Sugar Calories	10 almonds 0 Sugar Calories
LUNCH	Open-Faced Avocado Sandwich (see page 167) 65 Sugar Calories	Feta Pita Pizza (see page 170) 67 Sugar Calories	BLT Egg Sandwich (see page 169) 160 Sugar Calories
SNACK	1 string-cheese stick 0 Sugar Calories	1 hard-boiled egg 0 Sugar Calories	1 string-cheese stick 0 Sugar Calories
DINNER	Lasagna Cups (see page 175) 119 Sugar Calories	Spicy Corn Cakes (see page 173) 87 Sugar Calories	Zucchini Linguine (see page 176) 164 Sugar Calories
TREAT	Sweet Skinny Waffle (see page 217) 0 Sugar Calories	Sweet Skinny Waffle (see page 217) 0 Sugar Calories	Sweet Skinny Waffle (see page 217) 0 Sugar Calories
TOTAL	232 Sugar Calories	298 Sugar Calories	450 Sugar Calories

4 HAPPY	5 HAPPY	6 HAPPY	7 HAPPY
Tasty Toast & coffee with half-and-half (see page 146) 127 Sugar Calories	Ham and Egg Crepe Square & coffee with half-and-half (see page 143) 48 Sugar Calories	Peanut Butter and Strawberry Toasts & coffee with half-and-half (see page 145) 144 Sugar Calories	Baja Toast & coffee with half-and-half (see page 147) 126 Sugar Calories
¼ cup pumpkin seeds 0 Sugar Calories	10 almonds 0 Sugar Calories	¼ cup pumpkin seeds 0 Sugar Calories	10 almonds 0 Sugar Calories
Sweet Spinach Salad (see page 171) 139 Sugar Calories	Open-Faced Avocado Sandwich (see page 167) 65 Sugar Calories	Feta Pita Pizza (see page 170) 67 Sugar Calories	Sweet Spinach Salad (see page 171) 139 Sugar Calories
1 hard-boiled egg 0 Sugar Calories	1 string-cheese stick 0 Sugar Calories	1 hard-boiled egg 0 Sugar Calories	1 string-cheese stick 0 Sugar Calories
Catch of the Day (see page 177) 35 Sugar Calories	Lasagna Cups (see page 175) 119 Sugar Calories	Spicy Corn Cakes (see page 173) 87 Sugar Calories	Zucchini Linguine (see page 176) 164 Sugar Calories
Sweet Skinny Waffle (see page 217) 0 Sugar Calories	Sweet Skinny Waffle (see page 217) 0 Sugar Calories	Sweet Skinny Waffle (see page 217) 0 Sugar Calories	Sweet Skinny Waffle (see page 217) 0 Sugar Calories
301 Sugar Calories	232 Sugar Calories	298 Sugar Calories	429 Sugar Calories

extra-happy shopping list

PRODUCE

16-oz. package baby spinach

romaine lettuce

5 radishes

1 broccoli head, or package of chopped broccoli (at least 1 cup worth)

1 ear corn

1 tomato

1 large zucchini

2 avocados

1 carton strawberries

1 apple

1 pear

2 lemons

1 small red onion

1 head of garlic

parsley

fresh basil

MEAT/FISH

12 eggs

1 package bacon

1 oz. ground beef

1 halibut fillet

sliced deli ham

DAIRY

string-cheese sticks

pepper Jack cheese

Parmesan, grated

mozzarella, shredded

½ cup goat cheese, soft

¼ cup goat cheese, crumbles

feta cheese, crumbles

½ cup blue cheese, crumbles

2 slices provolone

1 cup ricotta cheese

2 Tbsp. cream cheese

2 tsp. buttermilk

half-and-half

whipping cream

butter

OTHER

I small baguette

8 slices whole-grain bread

2 slices pumpernickel bread

2 slices whole-wheat bread

I whole-wheat pita bread

I package small artisan rolls

I oz. chopped pecans

2 oz. almonds

4 oz. pumpkin seeds

¼ cup wild rice

¼ cup black or Greek olives, pitted and sliced

2 Tbsp. sun-dried tomatoes, packed in oil

¼ cup Alfredo sauce

½ cup marinara sauce, no sugar added

I Tbsp. sugar-free fruit spread

2 Tbsp. peanut butter

4 oz. linguine

12 wonton wrappers

½ cup flour

2 Tbsp. cornmeal

4 packets Truvia

stevia

olive oil

canola oil

coffee

salt

pepper

baking powder

baking soda

mayonnaise

7 Skinny Waffles™ (skinnywaffle.com)

Barlean's The Essential Woman Chocolate Mint Swirl

	1 HAPPY	2 HAPPY	3 HAPPY
BREAK-FAST	Maple Bacon Sandwich & coffee with half-and-half (see page 149) 80 Sugar Calories	Chicks on a Nest & coffee with half-and-half (see page 152) 120 Sugar Calories	Sunshine Wrap & coffee with half-and-half (see page 151) 42 Sugar Calories
SNACK	3 celery sticks spread with cream cheese 0 Sugar Calories	10 macadamia nuts 0 Sugar Calories	3 celery sticks spread with cream cheese 0 Sugar Calories
LUNCH	Heirloom Tomato Toasts (see page 179) 160 Sugar Calories	Rockin' Ravioli (see page 182) 100 Sugar Calories	Rice and Bean Stuffed Pepper (see page 181) 120 Sugar Calories
SNACK	1 string-cheese stick 0 Sugar Calories	1 slice deli turkey & 1 slice cheddar 0 Sugar Calories	1 string-cheese stick 0 Sugar Calories
DINNER	Sweet Potato Skins (see page 185) 79 Sugar Calories	Penne Marinara (see page 188) 156 Sugar Calories	Sautéed Scallops (see page 187) 72 Sugar Calories
TREAT	2-Minute Cake (see page 215) 0 Sugar Calories	2-Minute Cake (see page 215) 0 Sugar Calories	2-Minute Cake (see page 215) 0 Sugar Calories
TOTAL	319 Sugar Calories	376 Sugar Calories	234 Sugar Calories

4 HAPPY	5 HAPPY	6 HAPPY	7 HAPPY
Kale and Goat Cheese Scramble & coffee with half-and-half (see page 153) 60 Sugar Calories	Maple Bacon Sandwich & coffee with half-and-half (see page 149) 80 Sugar Calories	Chicks on a Nest & coffee with half-and-half (see page 152) 120 Sugar Calories	Sunshine Wrap & coffee with half-and-half (see page 151) 42 Sugar Calories
10 macadamia nuts 0 Sugar Calories	3 celery sticks spread with cream cheese 0 Sugar Calories	10 macadamia nuts 0 Sugar Calories	3 celery sticks spread with cream cheese 0 Sugar Calories
Prosciutto Wrap (see page 183) 80 Sugar Calories	Heirloom Tomato Toasts (see page 179) 160 Sugar Calories	Rockin' Ravioli (see page 182) 100 Sugar Calories	Rice and Bean Stuffed Pepper (see page 181) 120 Sugar Calories
1 slice deli turkey & 1 slice cheddar 0 Sugar Calories	1 string-cheese stick 0 Sugar Calories	1 slice deli turkey & 1 slice cheddar 0 Sugar Calories	1 string-cheese stick 0 Sugar Calories
Savory Kebab (see page 189) 90 Sugar Calories	Sweet Potato Skins (see page 185) 79 Sugar Calories	Penne Marinara (see page 188) 156 Sugar Calories	Sautéed Scallops (see page 187) 72 Sugar Calories
2-Minute Cake (see page 215) 0 Sugar Calories	2-Minute Cake (see page 215) 0 Sugar Calories	2-Minute Cake (see page 215) 0 Sugar Calories	2-Minute Cake (see page 215) 0 Sugar Calories
230 Sugar Calories	319 Sugar Calories	376 Sugar Calories	234 Sugar Calories

WEEK 2

extra-happy shopping list

PRODUCE

5½ cups spinach

½ cup arugula

½ cup alfalfa sprouts

1 cup kale

3 asparagus stalks

1 tomato (or 1 tomato
and 4 heirloom
tomatoes)

1 bunch celery

½ cup eggplant

1 cup broccoli

3 red bell peppers

2 potatoes

1 sweet potato

½ onion

2 Tbsp. chives

1 shallot

5 garlic gloves

2 Tbsp. fresh basil

MEAT/FISH

16 eggs

2 Italian sausages

6–12 scallops

6 slices maple bacon

3 oz. chicken

3 slices prosciutto

3 slices deli turkey

DAIRY

½ cup mozzarella

¾ cup goat cheese,
crumbled

¼ cup pepper Jack
cheese

½ cup feta cheese,
crumbled

7 slices cheddar
cheese

4 string-cheese sticks

2 Tbsp. sour cream

butter

half-and-half

whipping cream

cream cheese

Parmesan

OTHER

30 macadamia nuts

¼ cup pine nuts

1 small whole-grain baguette

5 slices whole-grain bread

1 package small artisan rolls

2 spinach tortilla wraps

1 whole-wheat wrap

10 whole-wheat cheese ravioli

4 oz. whole-wheat penne pasta

1 cup brown rice

½ cup black beans

¼ cup chickpeas

2 Tbsp. soy sauce

2 tsp. cumin

1 Tbsp. pesto

¼ cup marinara sauce, no sugar added

½ cup unsweetened cocoa powder

1 cup almond flour

½ cup Truvia Baking Blend

2 packets Truvia

baking powder

baking soda

olive oil

coconut oil

coffee

salt

pepper

	1 HAPPY	2 HAPPY	3 HAPPY
BREAK-FAST	Bacon Eggs Benedict & coffee with half-and-half (see page 155) 50 Sugar Calories	Ricotta Omelet & coffee with half-and-half (see page 158) 104 Sugar Calories	Nutty Oatmeal & coffee with half-and-half (see page 157) 120 Sugar Calories
SNACK	10 almonds 0 Sugar Calories	¼ cup sunflower seeds 0 Sugar Calories	10 almonds 0 Sugar Calories
LUNCH	Steak and Goat Cheese Quesadilla (see page 191) 127 Sugar Calories	Feta Turkey Burger (see page 194) 120 Sugar Calories	Spinach Pasta with Shrimp (see page 197) 53 Sugar Calories
SNACK	1 string-cheese stick 0 Sugar Calories	1 hard-boiled egg 0 Sugar Calories	1 string-cheese stick 0 Sugar Calories
DINNER	Sweet Kale Wrap (see page 193) 184 Sugar Calories	Citrus Shrimp (see page 195) 90 Sugar Calories	Italian Chicken Pita (see page 201) 150 Sugar Calories
TREAT	Sweet Skinny Waffle (see page 217) 0 Sugar Calories	Sweet Skinny Waffle (see page 217) 0 Sugar Calories	Sweet Skinny Waffle (see page 217) 0 Sugar Calories
TOTAL	361 Sugar Calories	314 Sugar Calories	323 Sugar Calories

4 HAPPY	5 HAPPY	6 HAPPY	7 HAPPY
Fruity Yogurt & coffee with half-and-half (see page 159) 33 Sugar Calories	Bacon Eggs Benedict & coffee with half-and-half (see page 155) 50 Sugar Calories	Ricotta Omelet & coffee with half-and-half (see page 158) 104 Sugar Calories	Nutty Oatmeal & coffee with half-and-half (see page 157) 120 Sugar Calories
¼ cup sunflower seeds 0 Sugar Calories	10 almonds 0 Sugar Calories	¼ cup sunflower seeds 0 Sugar Calories	10 almonds 0 Sugar Calories
Chicken Spanish Wrap (see page 200) 80 Sugar Calories	Steak and Goat Cheese Quesadilla (see page 191) 127 Sugar Calories	Feta Turkey Burger (see page 194) 120 Sugar Calories	Spinach Pasta with Shrimp (see page 197) 53 Sugar Calories
1 hard-boiled egg 0 Sugar Calories	1 string-cheese stick 0 Sugar Calories	1 hard-boiled egg 0 Sugar Calories	1 string-cheese stick 0 Sugar Calories
Bacon Spaghetti with Garlic Croutons (see page 199) 168 Sugar Calories	Sweet Kale Wrap (see page 193) 184 Sugar Calories	Citrus Shrimp (see page 195) 90 Sugar Calories	Italian Chicken Pita (see page 201) 150 Sugar Calories
Sweet Skinny Waffle (see page 217) 0 Sugar Calories	Sweet Skinny Waffle (see page 217) 0 Sugar Calories	Sweet Skinny Waffle (see page 217) 0 Sugar Calories	Sweet Skinny Waffle (see page 217) 0 Sugar Calories
281 Sugar Calories	361 Sugar Calories	314 Sugar Calories	323 Sugar Calories

extra-happy shopping list

PRODUCE

½ cup arugula	2 tsp. jalapeños	1 mango
1¾ cup spinach	½ cup kale	1 Tbsp. blackberries
1 cup mixed greens	2 Tbsp. mushrooms	1 Tbsp. blueberries
shredded lettuce	1 Tbsp. onion, chopped	1 garlic clove
¾ avocado		fresh cilantro
9 cherry tomatoes	1 red onion	fresh basil
1 Tbsp. tomato, chopped	1 lemon	fresh parsley
	2 limes	

MEAT/FISH

15 eggs	5 strips bacon	6 strips flank steak
18 medium shrimp	2 chicken breasts	2 turkey patties

DAIRY

1 Tbsp. cheddar cheese	4 slices provolone	whipping cream
	¼ cup goat cheese	half-and-half
4 string-cheese sticks	¼ cup feta cheese	butter
¼ cup ricotta cheese	¼ cup Greek yogurt	

OTHER

½ cup unsweetened vanilla almond milk

¼ cup unsweetened coconut flakes

3 English muffins

¾ cup whole-wheat spaghetti

5 garlic croutons

½ cup steel-cut oats

7 whole-wheat tortillas

2 whole-wheat hamburger buns

2 whole-wheat pitas

1½ cups spinach pasta

1 can black beans

1¼ cup brown rice

hummus

2 Tbsp. marinara sauce, no sugar added

2 Tbsp. mayonnaise

40 almonds

2 Tbsp. pecans

¾ cup sunflower seeds

2 Tbsp. walnuts

Truvia

stevia

olive oil

almond flour

cinnamon

red pepper flakes

red wine vinegar

balsamic vinegar

coffee

nonstick cooking spray

7 Skinny Waffles™ (skinnywaffle.com)

Barlean's The Essential Woman Chocolate Mint Swirl

	1 HAPPY	2 HAPPY	3 HAPPY
BREAK-FAST	Egg-in-a-Hole Sandwich & coffee with half-and-half (see page 161) 53 Sugar Calories	Fruit and Nut Yogurt & coffee with half-and-half (see page 164) 8 Sugar Calories	Baked Oatmeal Muffins & coffee with half-and-half (see page 163) 78 Sugar Calories
SNACK	3 celery sticks dipped in mustard 0 Sugar Calories	10 pecans 0 Sugar Calories	3 celery sticks dipped in mustard 0 Sugar Calories
LUNCH	Spinach Macaroni Bites (see page 203) 148 Sugar Calories	Chicken Stir-fry (see page 206) 99 Sugar Calories	Guacamole Grilled Cheese (see page 205) 120 Sugar Calories
SNACK	10 macadamia nuts 0 Sugar Calories	1 slice deli turkey & 1 slice cheddar cheese 0 Sugar Calories	10 macadamia nuts 0 Sugar Calories
DINNER	Spinach Bacon Quesadilla (see page 209) 82 Sugar Calories	Pesto Pita Pizza (see page 212) 70 Sugar Calories	Mediterranean Tacos (see page 211) 54 Sugar Calories
TREAT	2-Minute Cake (see page 215) 0 Sugar Calories	2-Minute Cake (see page 215) 0 Sugar Calories	2-Minute Cake (see page 215) 0 Sugar Calories
TOTAL	283 Sugar Calories	177 Sugar Calories	252 Sugar Calories

4 HAPPY	5 HAPPY	6 HAPPY	7 HAPPY
Ricotta Toast & coffee with half-and-half (see page 165) 102 Sugar Calories	Egg-in-a-Hole Sandwich & coffee with half-and-half (see page 161) 53 Sugar Calories	Fruit and Nut Yogurt & coffee with half-and-half (see page 164) 8 Sugar Calories	Baked Oatmeal Muffins & coffee with half-and-half (see page 163) 78 Sugar Calories
10 pecans 0 Sugar Calories	3 celery sticks dipped in mustard 0 Sugar Calories	10 pecans 0 Sugar Calories	3 celery sticks dipped in mustard 0 Sugar Calories
Pig in a Wrap (see page 207) 86 Sugar Calories	Spinach Macaroni Bites (see page 203) 148 Sugar Calories	Chicken Stir-fry (see page 206) 99 Sugar Calories	Guacamole Grilled Cheese (see page 205) 120 Sugar Calories
1 slice deli turkey & 1 slice cheddar cheese 0 Sugar Calories	10 macadamia nuts 0 Sugar Calories	1 slice deli turkey & 1 slice cheddar cheese 0 Sugar Calories	10 macadamia nuts 0 Sugar Calories
Tuna Melt (see page 213) 60 Sugar Calories	Spinach Bacon Quesadilla (see page 209) 82 Sugar Calories	Pesto Pita Pizza (see page 212) 70 Sugar Calories	Mediterranean Tacos (see page 211) 54 Sugar Calories
2-Minute Cake (see page 215) 0 Sugar Calories	2-Minute Cake (see page 215) 0 Sugar Calories	2-Minute Cake (see page 215) 0 Sugar Calories	2-Minute Cake (see page 215) 0 Sugar Calories
248 Sugar Calories	283 Sugar Calories	177 Sugar Calories	252 Sugar Calories

extra-happy shopping list

PRODUCE

3 cups spinach

½ cup shredded
  romaine

1 avocado

½ cup broccoli

½ carrot

1 bunch celery

½ cup onion,
  chopped

1 tomato

1 lemon

6 strawberries

2 bananas

2 cups blueberries

1 Tbsp. ginger

2 garlic cloves

fresh basil

MEAT/FISH

8 eggs

2 fillets mahi mahi

½ can tuna

6 strips bacon

2 slices Canadian
  bacon

4 chicken breasts

3 slices deli turkey

DAIRY

2 tsp. Parmesan
  cheese

2 Tbsp. ricotta cheese

cheddar cheese
  (11 slices and 2
  Tbsp. shredded)

mozzarella cheese

¼ cup feta cheese

½ cup plain
  Greek yogurt

2 Tbsp. cream cheese

butter

half-and-half

whipping cream

OTHER

- 2 slices whole-wheat bread
- 5 slices whole-grain bread
- 1 whole-wheat English muffin
- 4 small corn tortillas
- 3 whole-wheat tortillas (wraps)
- 1 whole-wheat pita
- 2 cups macaroni noodles
- 1 cup rice
- 7 cups oats
- ¼ cup almonds

- 40 macadamia nuts
- 30 pecans
- ½ cup ground flaxseed
- ½ cup unsweetened cocoa powder
- 3 cups unsweetened applesauce
- 2 Tbsp. black olives
- 2 tsp. pesto
- ¼ cup pico de gallo
- 2 Tbsp. salsa
- 2 Tbsp. sugar-free preserves
- 2 tsp. vanilla extract

- 8 packets stevia
- 4 packets Truvia
- ½ cup Truvia Baking Blend
- baking powder
- baking soda
- almond flour
- coconut oil
- olive oil
- mayonnaise
- mustard
- cinnamon
- coffee

	1 SLIM	2 SLIM	3 SLIM
BREAK-FAST	Breakfast Lasagna & coffee with half-and-half (see page 109) 0 Sugar Calories	Breakfast Shake & coffee with half-and-half (see page 112) 0 Sugar Calories	Breakfast Lasagna & coffee with half-and-half (see page 109) 0 Sugar Calories
SNACK	10 almonds 0 Sugar Calories	¼ cup pumpkin seeds 0 Sugar Calories	10 almonds 0 Sugar Calories
LUNCH	Chicken Salad–Stuffed Tomatoes (see page 121) 0 Sugar Calories	Tuna Cups (see page 124) 0 Sugar Calories	Chicken Salad–Stuffed Tomatoes (see page 121) 0 Sugar Calories
SNACK	1 string-cheese stick 0 Sugar Calories	1 hard-boiled egg 0 Sugar Calories	1 string-cheese stick 0 Sugar Calories
DINNER	Italian Salad (see page 125) 0 Sugar Calories	Eggplant Rollups (see page 123) 0 Sugar Calories	Italian Salad (see page 125) 0 Sugar Calories
TREAT	2-Minute Cake (see page 215) 0 Sugar Calories	2-Minute Cake (see page 215) 0 Sugar Calories	2-Minute Cake (see page 215) 0 Sugar Calories
TOTAL	0 Sugar Calories	0 Sugar Calories	0 Sugar Calories

If you find that you are super motivated, energetic, positive, and enthusiastic—and Sugar Calories are not calling your name—give the Extra-Slim Plan a go. On this food plan, you'll eat limited Sugar Calories all week long. Just remember that if your mood begins to drop at any time, you can switch to the standard Carb Cycling Plan or even the Extra-Happy Plan—just aim for at least 2 Slim Days most weeks.

4 SLIM	5 SLIM	6 SLIM	7 SLIM
Breakfast Shake & coffee with half-and-half (see page 112) 0 Sugar Calories	Breakfast Lasagna & coffee with half-and-half (see page 109) 0 Sugar Calories	Breakfast Shake & coffee with half-and-half (see page 112) 0 Sugar Calories	Breakfast Lasagna & coffee with half-and-half (see page 109) 0 Sugar Calories
¼ cup pumpkin seeds 0 Sugar Calories	10 almonds 0 Sugar Calories	¼ cup pumpkin seeds 0 Sugar Calories	10 almonds 0 Sugar Calories
Tuna Cups (see page 124) 0 Sugar Calories	Chicken Salad–Stuffed Tomatoes (see page 121) 0 Sugar Calories	Tuna Cups (see page 124) 0 Sugar Calories	Chicken Salad–Stuffed Tomatoes (see page 121) 0 Sugar Calories
1 hard-boiled egg 0 Sugar Calories	1 string-cheese stick 0 Sugar Calories	1 hard-boiled egg 0 Sugar Calories	1 string-cheese stick 0 Sugar Calories
Eggplant Rollups (see page 123) 0 Sugar Calories	Italian Salad (see page 125) 0 Sugar Calories	Eggplant Rollups (see page 123) 0 Sugar Calories	Italian Salad (see page 125) 0 Sugar Calories
2-Minute Cake (see page 215) 0 Sugar Calories	2-Minute Cake (see page 215) 0 Sugar Calories	2-Minute Cake (see page 215) 0 Sugar Calories	2-Minute Cake (see page 215) 0 Sugar Calories
0 Sugar Calories	0 Sugar Calories	0 Sugar Calories	0 Sugar Calories

WEEK 1

extra-slim shopping list

PRODUCE

9 whole romaine leaves

8 cups shredded
   romaine

4 yellow zucchinis, large

1 cup mushrooms,
   chopped

½ cup broccoli,
   chopped

1 zucchini

1 avocado

4 tomatoes

20 cherry tomatoes

2 scallions

3 eggplants, large

4 limes

½ cup red onion,
   chopped

1½ cups onion,
   chopped

fresh basil

cilantro

parsley

MEAT/FISH

10 eggs

16 oz. breakfast
   sausage

2 cups chicken,
   shredded

4 cups chicken, sliced

3 cans tuna

16 slices pepperoni

DAIRY

4 string cheese sticks

¾ cup ricotta

¾ cup Parmesan,
   grated

half-and-half

whipping cream

OTHER

40 almonds

¾ cup pumpkin seeds

1 jar marinara sauce,
no sugar added

2 packets Truvia

stevia

unsweetened coconut
milk

Strawberry Jay Robb
whey protein

olive oil

coffee

garlic powder

onion powder

cumin

chili powder

salt

pepper

dried oregano

dried basil

mayonnaise

7 Skinny Waffles™
(skinnywaffle.com)

Barlean's The Essential
Woman Chocolate
Mint Swirl

WEEK 2: EXTRA-SLIM MEAL PLANNER

	1 SLIM	2 SLIM	3 SLIM
BREAK-FAST	Traditional Skinny Waffle & coffee with half-and-half (see page 111) 0 Sugar Calories	Breakfast Shake & coffee with half-and-half (see page 112) 0 Sugar Calories	Traditional Skinny Waffle & coffee with half-and-half (see page 111) 0 Sugar Calories
SNACK	3 celery sticks spread with cream cheese 0 Sugar Calories	10 macadamia nuts 0 Sugar Calories	3 celery sticks spread with cream cheese 0 Sugar Calories
LUNCH	Classic Wedge Salad (see page 127) 0 Sugar Calories	Italian Salad (see page 125) 0 Sugar Calories	Classic Wedge Salad (see page 127) 0 Sugar Calories
SNACK	1 string-cheese stick 0 Sugar Calories	1 slice deli turkey & 1 slice cheddar 0 Sugar Calories	1 string-cheese stick 0 Sugar Calories
DINNER	Basil Pesto Pizza (see page 129) 0 Sugar Calories	Turkey Caesar Salad (see page 130) 0 Sugar Calories	Basil Pesto Pizza (see page 129) 0 Sugar Calories
TREAT	2-Minute Cake (see page 215) 0 Sugar Calories	2-Minute Cake (see page 215) 0 Sugar Calories	2-Minute Cake (see page 215) 0 Sugar Calories
TOTAL	0 Sugar Calories	0 Sugar Calories	0 Sugar Calories

4 SLIM	5 SLIM	6 SLIM	7 SLIM
Breakfast Shake & coffee with half-and-half (see page 112) 0 Sugar Calories	Traditional Skinny Waffle & coffee with half-and-half (see page 111) 0 Sugar Calories	Breakfast Shake & coffee with half-and-half (see page 112) 0 Sugar Calories	Traditional Skinny Waffle & coffee with half-and-half (see page 111) 0 Sugar Calories
10 macadamia nuts 0 Sugar Calories	3 celery sticks spread with cream cheese 0 Sugar Calories	10 macadamia nuts 0 Sugar Calories	3 celery sticks spread with cream cheese 0 Sugar Calories
Italian Salad (see page 125) 0 Sugar Calories	Classic Wedge Salad (see page 127) 0 Sugar Calories	Italian Salad (see page 125) 0 Sugar Calories	Classic Wedge Salad (see page 127) 0 Sugar Calories
1 slice deli turkey & 1 slice cheddar 0 Sugar Calories	1 string-cheese stick 0 Sugar Calories	1 slice deli turkey & 1 slice cheddar 0 Sugar Calories	1 string-cheese stick 0 Sugar Calories
Turkey Caesar Salad (see page 130) 0 Sugar Calories	Basil Pesto Pizza (see page 129) 0 Sugar Calories	Turkey Caesar Salad (see page 130) 0 Sugar Calories	Basil Pesto Pizza (see page 129) 0 Sugar Calories
2-Minute Cake (see page 215) 0 Sugar Calories	2-Minute Cake (see page 215) 0 Sugar Calories	2-Minute Cake (see page 215) 0 Sugar Calories	2-Minute Cake (see page 215) 0 Sugar Calories
0 Sugar Calories	0 Sugar Calories	0 Sugar Calories	0 Sugar Calories

extra-slim shopping list

PRODUCE

2 heads iceberg lettuce

9 cups shredded romaine

2 heads cauliflower

1 bunch celery

½ cup red onion, chopped

½ cup broccoli, chopped

½ cup tomato, chopped

15 cherry tomatoes

1 tsp. garlic

¼ cup fresh basil

MEAT/FISH

12 eggs

12 slices pepperoni

8 strips bacon

3 slices deli turkey

1 cup turkey, shredded

3 cups chicken, sliced

DAIRY

¾ cup Parmesan

½ cup blue cheese, crumbled

3 slices cheddar cheese

4 string-cheese sticks

3 cups mozzarella

half-and-half

whipping cream

cream cheese

butter

OTHER

½ cup blue cheese dressing, no sugar added

½ cup Caesar dressing

½ cup marinara, no sugar added

1 cup pesto

1 cup almond flour

½ cup unsweetened cocoa powder

½ cup Truvia Baking Blend

2 packets Truvia

unsweetened almond milk

Jay Robb vanilla whey protein

baking powder

baking soda

dried oregano

garlic salt

dried basil

olive oil

coconut oil

coffee

salt

pepper

4 Skinny Waffles™ (skinnywaffle.com)

Skinny Maple Syrup™ (skinnymaplesyrup.com)

WEEK 3: EXTRA-SLIM MEAL PLANNER

	1 SLIM	2 SLIM	3 SLIM
BREAK-FAST	Sautéed Vegetable Frittata & coffee with half-and-half (see page 115) 0 Sugar Calories	Cinnamon-Nut Cottage Cheese & coffee with half-and-half (see page 118) 0 Sugar Calories	Sautéed Vegetable Frittata & coffee with half-and-half (see page 115) 0 Sugar Calories
SNACK	10 almonds 0 Sugar Calories	¼ cup sunflower seeds 0 Sugar Calories	10 almonds 0 Sugar Calories
LUNCH	Chicken Caprese Stacks (see page 133) 0 Sugar Calories	Dijon Salmon (see page 131) 0 Sugar Calories	Chicken Caprese Stacks (see page 133) 0 Sugar Calories
SNACK	1 string-cheese stick 0 Sugar Calories	1 hard-boiled egg 0 Sugar Calories	1 string-cheese stick 0 Sugar Calories
DINNER	Zucchini Boats (see page 135) 0 Sugar Calories	Steak Kebab (see page 136) 0 Sugar Calories	Zucchini Boats (see page 135) 0 Sugar Calories
TREAT	Sweet Skinny Waffle (see page 217) 0 Sugar Calories	Sweet Skinny Waffle (see page 217) 0 Sugar Calories	Sweet Skinny Waffle (see page 217) 0 Sugar Calories
TOTAL	0 Sugar Calories	0 Sugar Calories	0 Sugar Calories

4 SLIM	5 SLIM	6 SLIM	7 SLIM
Cinnamon-Nut Cottage Cheese & coffee with half-and-half (see page 118) 0 Sugar Calories	Sautéed Vegetable Frittata & coffee with half-and-half (see page 115) 0 Sugar Calories	Cinnamon-Nut Cottage Cheese & coffee with half-and-half (see page 118) 0 Sugar Calories	Sautéed Vegetable Frittata & coffee with half-and-half (see page 115) 0 Sugar Calories
¼ cup sunflower seeds 0 Sugar Calories	10 almonds 0 Sugar Calories	¼ cup sunflower seeds 0 Sugar Calories	10 almonds 0 Sugar Calories
Dijon Salmon (see page 131) 0 Sugar Calories	Chicken Caprese Stacks (see page 133) 0 Sugar Calories	Dijon Salmon (see page 131) 0 Sugar Calories	Chicken Caprese Stacks (see page 133) 0 Sugar Calories
1 hard-boiled egg 0 Sugar Calories	1 string-cheese stick 0 Sugar Calories	1 hard-boiled egg 0 Sugar Calories	1 string-cheese stick 0 Sugar Calories
Steak Kebab (see page 136) 0 Sugar Calories	Zucchini Boats (see page 135) 0 Sugar Calories	Steak Kebab (see page 136) 0 Sugar Calories	Zucchini Boats (see page 135) 0 Sugar Calories
Sweet Skinny Waffle (see page 217) 0 Sugar Calories	Sweet Skinny Waffle (see page 217) 0 Sugar Calories	Sweet Skinny Waffle (see page 217) 0 Sugar Calories	Sweet Skinny Waffle (see page 217) 0 Sugar Calories
0 Sugar Calories	0 Sugar Calories	0 Sugar Calories	0 Sugar Calories

extra-slim shopping list

PRODUCE

5½ cups spinach

13 asparagus stalks

1 red bell pepper

16 cherry tomatoes

1 cup mushrooms

1 red onion

3 onions

3 tomatoes

2 zucchinis

fresh basil

MEAT/FISH

11 eggs

2 salmon fillets

9 oz. steak

4 chicken breasts

12 slices bacon

DAIRY

4 string-cheese sticks

4 slices mozzarella

½ cup cheddar cheese

1½ cups cottage cheese

¼ cup sour cream

half-and-half

whipping cream

OTHER

3 Tbsp. Dijon mustard

40 almonds

½ cup pecans

¾ cup sunflower seeds

2 packets Truvia

stevia

olive oil

red wine vinegar

balsamic vinegar

cinnamon

curry powder

thyme

pepper

salt

coffee

7 Skinny Waffles™ (skinnywaffle.com)

Barlean's The Essential Woman Chocolate Mint Swirl

QUICK TIPS FOR STAYING ON TRACK

- Review your planner before the week begins.

- Make ahead: If you notice that you'll be having a snack more than once, then prep a batch on Sunday so you have them on hand all week.

- Prepackage for easy on-the-go: Take a few moments to throw the nuts you'll be eating for a snack into sandwich bags so you'll have them ready when you run out the door. Ditto for celery sticks.

- Don't get caught hungry: Stash a few baggies of nuts in your work desk or in your car, so you don't head to the vending machine or fast-food joint when you get hungry.

	1 SLIM	2 SLIM	3 SLIM
BREAK-FAST	Poached Prosciutto & coffee with half-and-half (see page 117) 0 Sugar Calories	Nutty Cottage Cheese & coffee with half-and-half (see page 119) 0 Sugar Calories	Poached Prosciutto & coffee with half-and-half (see page 117) 0 Sugar Calories
SNACK	3 celery sticks dipped in mustard 0 Sugar Calories	10 pecans 0 Sugar Calories	3 celery sticks dipped in mustard 0 Sugar Calories
LUNCH	Jalapeño Bites (see page 139) 0 Sugar Calories	Green Greek Salad (see page 137) 0 Sugar Calories	Jalapeño Bites (see page 139) 0 Sugar Calories
SNACK	10 macadamia nuts 0 Sugar Calories	1 slice deli turkey & 1 slice cheddar cheese 0 Sugar Calories	10 macadamia nuts 0 Sugar Calories
DINNER	Stuffed Salmon (see page 141) 0 Sugar Calories	Tuna Cups (see page 124) 0 Sugar Calories	Stuffed Salmon (see page 1141) 0 Sugar Calories
TREAT	2-Minute Cake (see page 215) 0 Sugar Calories	2-Minute Cake (see page 215) 0 Sugar Calories	2-Minute Cake (see page 215) 0 Sugar Calories
TOTAL	0 Sugar Calories	0 Sugar Calories	0 Sugar Calories

4 SLIM	5 SLIM	6 SLIM	7 SLIM
Nutty Cottage Cheese & coffee with half-and-half (see page 119) 0 Sugar Calories	Poached Prosciutto & coffee with half-and-half (see page 117) 0 Sugar Calories	Nutty Cottage Cheese & coffee with half-and-half (see page 119) 0 Sugar Calories	Poached Prosciutto & coffee with half-and-half (see page 117) 0 Sugar Calories
10 pecans 0 Sugar Calories	3 celery sticks dipped in mustard 0 Sugar Calories	10 pecans 0 Sugar Calories	3 celery sticks dipped in mustard 0 Sugar Calories
Green Greek Salad (see page 137) 0 Sugar Calories	Jalapeño Bites (see page 139) 0 Sugar Calories	Green Greek Salad (see page 137) 0 Sugar Calories	Jalapeño Bites (see page 139) 0 Sugar Calories
1 slice deli turkey & 1 slice cheddar cheese 0 Sugar Calories	10 macadamia nuts 0 Sugar Calories	1 slice deli turkey & 1 slice cheddar cheese 0 Sugar Calories	10 macadamia nuts 0 Sugar Calories
Tuna Cups (see page 124) 0 Sugar Calories	Stuffed Salmon (see page 141) 0 Sugar Calories	Tuna Cups (see page 124) 0 Sugar Calories	Stuffed Salmon (see page 141) 0 Sugar Calories
2-Minute Cake (see page 215) 0 Sugar Calories	2-Minute Cake (see page 215) 0 Sugar Calories	2-Minute Cake (see page 215) 0 Sugar Calories	2-Minute Cake (see page 215) 0 Sugar Calories
0 Sugar Calories	0 Sugar Calories	0 Sugar Calories	0 Sugar Calories

WEEK 4

extra-slim shopping list

PRODUCE

6 cups arugula

6 romaine leaves

2 cups spinach

3½ avocados

1 bunch celery

15 cherry tomatoes

3 tomatoes

1½ cucumbers

fresh dill

8 jalapeño peppers

½ cup red onion, chopped

3 lemons

2 garlic cloves

lime juice

fresh cilantro

MEAT/FISH

10 eggs

3 cans tuna

3 salmon fillets

3 slices deli turkey

16 slices prosciutto

16 strips bacon

3 chicken breasts

DAIRY

2 slices cheddar cheese

1½ cups cottage cheese

¼ cup cream cheese

½ cup feta cheese

¼ cup goat cheese

½ cup Parmesan cheese

¼ cup ricotta cheese

half-and-half

whipping cream

OTHER

15 Kalamata olives

½ cup almonds

40 macadamia nuts

30 pecans

½ cup unsweetened cocoa powder

½ cup Truvia Baking Blend

2 packets Truvia

coconut oil

olive oil

almond flour

baking powder

baking soda

white vinegar

red wine vinegar

1 cup quinoa

mustard

oregano

salt

pepper

coffee

nonstick cooking spray

16 toothpicks

recipe list

5

recipes

The honest truth is that I am busy, as I'm sure you are. To keep things easy for me, for the most part I stick to simple meals I know I can make. That being said, I do like to be in the kitchen, making things for friends and family. There is nothing like a homemade meal that fills the house with delicious aromas and tastes that make you feel alive.

The following are all featured in the meal planners each week and range from quick toss-together meals to more in-volved recipes. If there is a recipe you are not a fan of, it is completely fine to swap it for one you do like. Just make sure that you swap a Slim recipe for a Slim, and Happy for Happy. Enjoy!

MOST RECIPES SERVE ONE

Unless otherwise discussed, all the recipes below are made to serve one person; however, they are easily doubled or quadrupled depending on your needs. Don't stress about exact measurements, and keep in mind that I've designed these recipes to work well with a tad more or a tad less of an ingredient, especially when it is a Freebie. These are also great recipes to improvise with by substituting different vegetables based on your preferences or dietary sensitivities.

CODING FOR DIETARY SENSITIVITIES

Where applicable I've included a substitution list for vegetarians and vegans, as well as dairy-free, gluten-free, and seafood-free options. Look for these codes below the recipes to see suggestions:

VEGETARIAN = VEG   DAIRY-FREE = D   SEAFOOD-FREE = S
VEGAN = VGN   GLUTEN-FREE = G

SLIM DAYS RECIPES

Note: Feel free to add coffee with half-and-half to any breakfast choice.

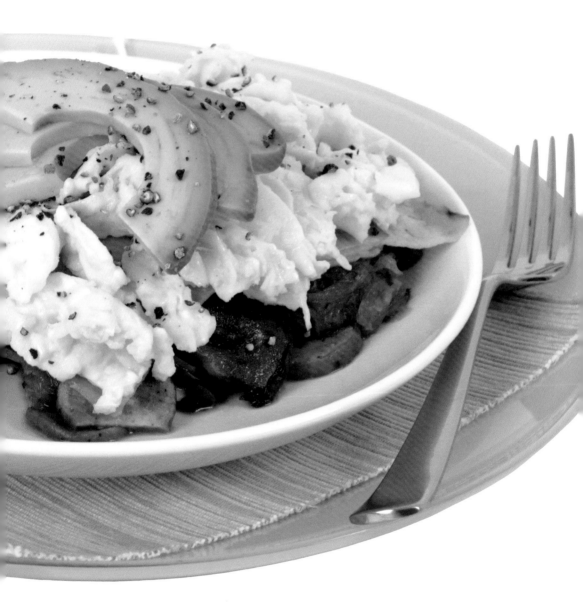

breakfast lasagna

0 SUGAR CALORIES, not 476 calories

Olive oil

¼ cup onions, chopped

¼ cup mushrooms, chopped

1 yellow zucchini, sliced thinly lengthwise

4 oz. cooked breakfast sausage, or 3 slices cooked bacon

1 Tbsp. of half-and-half

¼ tsp. garlic powder

¼ tsp. onion powder

1 egg

¼ sliced avocado

Nonstick cooking spray

Salt and pepper

QUICK TIP

You can buy frozen cooked breakfast sausage at the supermarket and heat it quickly in the microwave. Already-cooked bacon strips can be found in most grocery stores, to make this recipe extra-fast and cleanup a snap. If you are using uncooked bacon, sauté it first in the cast-iron skillet, and use a bit of the leftover bacon fat for your onion/mushroom sauté instead of olive oil. If you choose to skip the meat (vegetarian option) use two eggs instead of one.

Preheat oven to 375°F. Heat a cast-iron skillet on medium-high, add a tablespoon or two of olive oil for about a minute, then add the onions and mushrooms.

Turn the heat to medium and sauté for about 10 minutes, stirring frequently. In a small glass baking dish sprayed with nonstick cooking spray, layer sliced zucchini so it covers the bottom. Top it with the sautéed veggies, then layer with the meat. In a glass mixing cup, whisk together the half-and-half, garlic powder, and onion powder, then pour mixture over ingredients in baking dish. Sprinkle with salt and pepper, and put in oven for 30 to 32 minutes. When the "lasagna" is nearing the end of its cooking, scramble one or two eggs in the cast-iron skillet (add a bit more olive oil if needed). Serve the "lasagna" topped with the egg and sliced avocado.

VEG   use Quorn Bacon-Style Strips instead of sausage or bacon, or increase the egg to 2 eggs

VGN   omit egg, or substitute mashed firm tofu sautéed with ¼ tsp. turmeric; use Quorn Bacon-style strips instead of sausage or bacon; use unsweetened almond milk instead of half-and-half

D   omit half-and-half and increase eggs to two

G   yes

S   yes

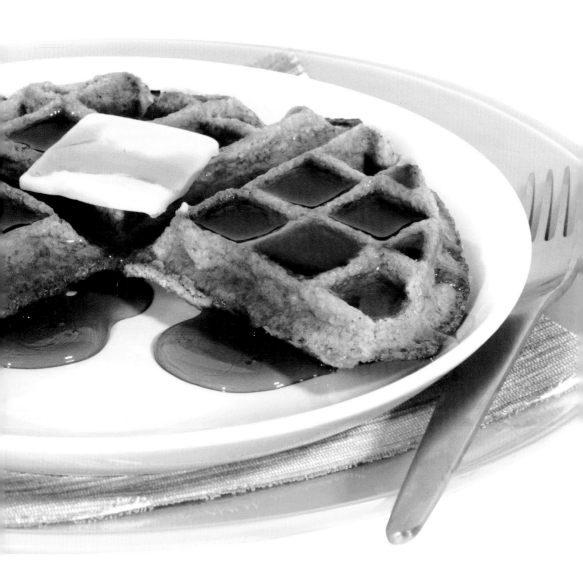

traditional skinny waffle

0 SUGAR CALORIES, not 546 calories

You can go to www.skinnywaffle.com to purchase these premade, no–Sugar Calorie waffles. Pop them in the toaster, top with butter and Skinny Maple Syrup (www.skinnymaplesyrup.com), and serve.

Additional, no–Sugar Calorie toppings to try:

- whipped cream
- cinnamon
- unsweetened cocoa powder
- nuts (pecans, pistachios, etc.)

Want to make them yourself? Here's how:

¼ cup coconut flour

1 Tbsp. unsweetened almond milk

2 tsp. cinnamon

1 Tbsp. Truvia Baking Blend

¼ tsp. baking powder

¼ tsp. sea salt

1 Tbsp. coconut oil

4 eggs

Nonstick cooking spray

Preheat waffle iron. Mix all ingredients well in a bowl. Spray waffle iron with cooking spray, then pour half the batter into the warm iron. Cook until golden brown. Remove from iron, and repeat with remaining batter.

breakfast shake

0 SUGAR CALORIES, not 160 calories

1 scoop Strawberry Jay Robb whey protein
1 cup unsweetened coconut milk

Shake, stir, or blend the whey protein powder and the coconut milk until well mixed.
Pour and serve.

QUICK TIP

If you feel like you need a
good mood boost,
add a mashed banana,
and mix up your shake
in a blender with a
few ice cubes.

VEG yes

VGN yes

D yes

G yes

S yes

vanilla breakfast shake

0 SUGAR CALORIES, not 110 calories

1 scoop Jay Robb vanilla whey protein
1 cup unsweetened almond milk (can also use water, but won't be as filling)

Shake, stir, or blend the whey protein powder and the almond milk until well mixed. Pour and serve.

QUICK TIP

Get nutty. You can also add a handful of almonds into the blender, or nosh on nuts on the side for a little extra energy.

VEG yes

VGN yes

D yes

G yes

S yes

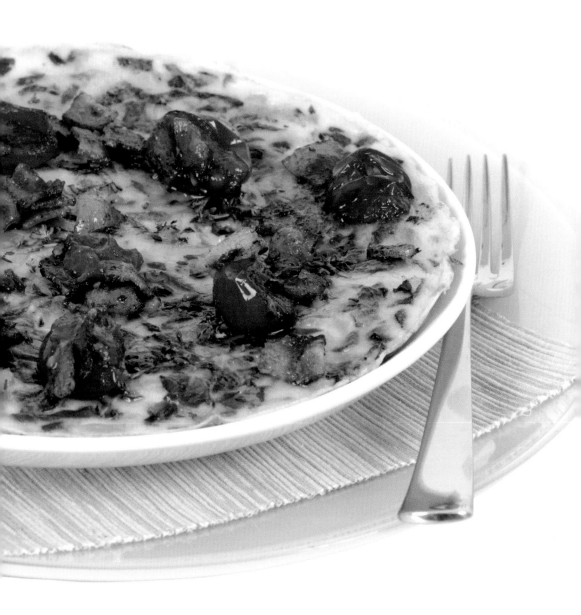

sautéed vegetable frittata

0 SUGAR CALORIES, not 309 calories

1 cup spinach, chopped

¼ cup mushrooms, chopped

¼ cup onions, chopped

1 asparagus stalk, white stem trimmed, and chopped

2 eggs

4 cherry tomatoes, cut in half

2 slices bacon

Salt and pepper

Preheat oven to 375°F. Heat a cast-iron or nonstick ovenproof skillet, and cook bacon according to package directions; remove and drain on paper towels. Reserve a tablespoon or two of the grease, and heat on medium-high. When hot, add the onions and mushrooms, stirring frequently until the onions are soft and the mushrooms release then reabsorb their liquid, about 5–10 minutes. Add the asparagus stalk and sauté for another 2 minutes, then add spinach and stir frequently, until spinach is just wilted, about 1 or 2 minutes.

Whisk the eggs in a bowl. When the vegetables are done, turn off the burner and stir in the eggs until just mixed, then season with salt and pepper. Eggs will cook a little. Put skillet in oven, and heat until the eggs are cooked through, 5–10 minutes. Serve topped with tomatoes and crumbled bacon.

QUICK TIP

For on-the-go options during the week, make extras of this recipe and freeze the leftovers. Just add the bacon and the tomatoes to the egg mixture and cook all together. To reheat, put in microwave for 1–2 minutes.

VEG   replace bacon with Lightlife Smart Bacon

VGN choose another option

D   yes

G   use Boar's Head Bacon

S   yes

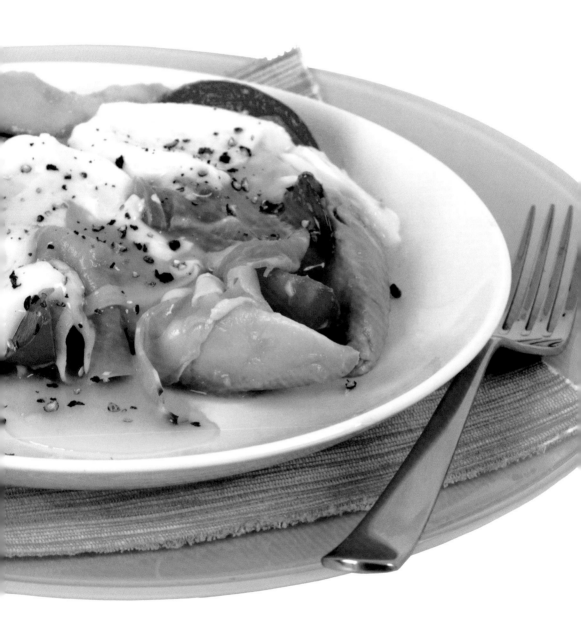

poached prosciutto

0 SUGAR CALORIES, not 360 calories

2 eggs

2 tsp. white vinegar

4 slices prosciutto

½ avocado, sliced

½ tomato, sliced

1 tsp. Parmesan cheese

Salt and pepper

Fill a small shallow saucepan with about 2" of water, and heat to almost boiling, and then add 1 or 2 tsp. vinegar (vinegar will help the egg whites congeal). Crack one of the eggs into a small cup, then place the cup near the edge of the hot water and gently pour into water; repeat with the other egg. You can use a spoon to help push the whites closer to the yolks—it helps hold them together. Turn off the heat, cover the pan, and let sit for 4 minutes until egg whites are cooked.

On a plate, layer the prosciutto, avocado, tomatoes, and then the eggs. Garnish with Parmesan, and adjust the salt and pepper seasoning to your liking.

QUICK TIP

One trick to make the eggs stay somewhat contained is to take a ring from a Mason jar and place it in the pan. Drop the egg over the Mason-jar ring and let it settle, then turn off the heat, cover the pan, and let sit for 4 minutes.

VEG   replace prosciutto with spinach leaves

VGN   choose another option

D   replace Parmesan with Daiya Mozzarella Style Shreds

G   yes

S   yes

cinnamon-nut cottage cheese

0 SUGAR CALORIES, not 240 calories

½ cup cottage cheese

2 Tbsp. chopped pecans

Dash of cinnamon

Put cottage cheese in a bowl, and top with nuts and a sprinkle of cinnamon.

QUICK TIP

This is also great topped with chopped walnuts, almonds, or macadamia nuts.

VEG yes

VGN omit cottage cheese, use mashed soft or silken tofu with a pinch of salt

D omit cottage cheese, use mashed soft or silken tofu with a pinch of salt

G yes

S yes

nutty cottage cheese

0 SUGAR CALORIES, not 240 calories

½ cup cottage cheese
2 Tbsp. sliced almonds

Put cottage cheese in a bowl and top with sliced almonds.

QUICK TIP

Add a sprinkle of cinnamon and 1 Tbsp. unsweetened coconut flakes for added flavor. You can also use chopped walnuts in place of the almonds.

VEG yes

VGN omit cottage cheese, use mashed soft or silken tofu with a pinch of salt

D omit cottage cheese, use mashed soft or silken tofu with a pinch of salt

G yes

S yes

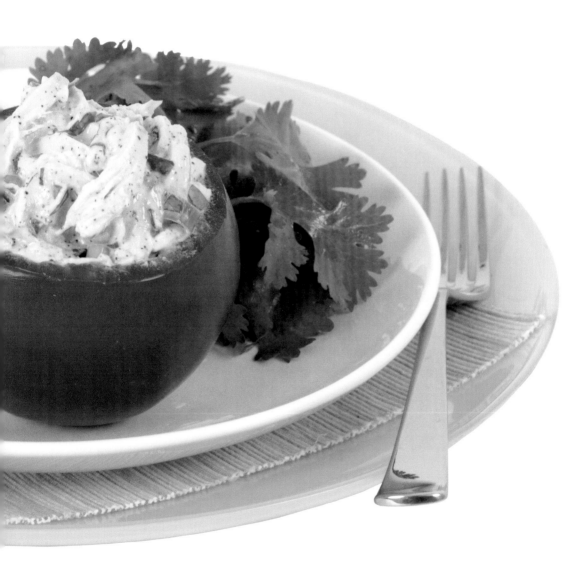

chicken salad–stuffed tomatoes

0 SUGAR CALORIES, not 230 calories

I hollowed-out tomato

½ cup cooked chicken, shredded

2 Tbsp. mayonnaise

½ sliced scallion

I Tbsp. chopped cilantro

I tsp. lime juice

Pinch garlic powder

Pinch cumin

Pinch chili powder

Salt and pepper to taste

In a small bowl, mix chicken, mayo, scallion, cilantro, lime juice, garlic powder, cumin, chili powder, and salt and pepper to taste. Fill tomato with chicken mixture.

VEG omit chicken and use Quorn Naked Chik'n Cutlet

VGN omit chicken and use Quorn Naked Chik'n Cutlet; omit mayonnaise and use Vegenaise

D yes

G use Heinz mayonnaise

S yes

QUICK TIP

For easy prep, use rotisserie chicken from the grocery store. You can also stock some canned chicken on your pantry shelf so that you can make this recipe even when you don't have time to run to the store for a cooked chicken.

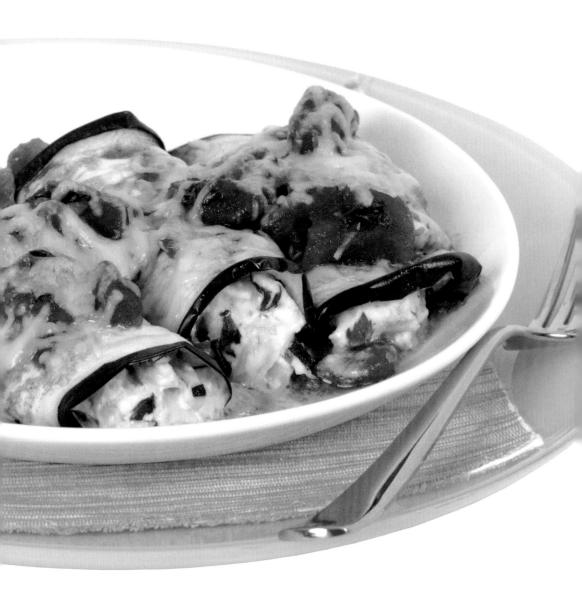

eggplant rollups

0 SUGAR CALORIES, not 231 calories

3 slices of a large eggplant, sliced lengthwise about ½" thick

Olive oil

2 Tbsp. chopped onion

¼ chopped zucchini

¼ cup ricotta

2 Tbsp. chopped parsley

1 tsp. chopped fresh basil

1 Tbsp. grated Parmesan cheese, and extra for garnish

1 egg

Salt and pepper

½ cup marinara sauce (no sugar added)

Preheat oven to 450°F. Brush the eggplant with oil and place on an oiled cookie sheet. Bake for 20 minutes. While the eggplant is in the oven, heat a skillet and add a little oil. Sauté the onion and zucchini for about 5 minutes (until just soft), then remove from heat. In a small bowl, mix together the onion, zucchini, ricotta, parsley, basil, Parmesan, egg, and salt and pepper. When eggplant is done, let cool slightly, then place equal amounts of cheese mixture in the middle of each roll. Roll the eggplant around the mixture, then place seam-side down in a small glass baking dish. Top each roll with marinara sauce and bake for 20 minutes, or until cheese has melted. Serve with Parmesan cheese sprinkled on top.

QUICK TIP

No ricotta on hand? You can use cottage cheese as a substitute. If you are out of Parmesan, feta cheese makes a good swap.

VEG yes

VGN omit Parmesan; replace ricotta with mashed tofu or Tofutti Better than Ricotta Cheese

D omit Parmesan; replace ricotta with mashed tofu or Tofutti Better than Ricotta Cheese

G yes

S yes

tuna cups

0 SUGAR CALORIES, not 353 calories

1 can tuna, drained
½ avocado
1 Tbsp. mayonnaise
1 lime
3 romaine leaves
Salt and pepper to taste

In a small bowl mash the avocado; then mix with tuna, mayo, juice from the lime, and salt and pepper to taste.

Serve on romaine leaves or on some shredded romaine lettuce.

VEG substitute mashed tofu in place of tuna

VGN substitute mashed tofu in place of tuna; omit mayonnaise and use Vegenaise

D yes

G yes

S substitute mashed tofu or canned chicken in place of tuna

QUICK TIP

Pump up your antioxidants and turn your cups into a salad. Instead of serving the tuna on top of romaine lettuce leaves, fill a bowl with baby spinach, baby arugula, and sliced red bell peppers, and top with the mixed tuna. Squeeze extra lime on top.

italian salad

0 SUGAR CALORIES, not 231 calories

2 cups romaine lettuce, shredded

½–1 cup cooked chicken, sliced

5 cherry tomatoes, sliced

2 Tbsp. chopped broccoli

2 Tbsp. sliced red onion

2 Tbsp. marinara sauce (no sugar added)

2 tsp. dried oregano

2 tsp. dried or fresh basil

4 slices pepperoni

2 Tbsp. Parmesan

Put a small pot of water on to boil. While your water is heating, prepare your veggies. When the water boils, drop in the broccoli until just tender crisp (about 5 minutes), and strain. Put the romaine, chicken, tomatoes, onion, and broccoli in a medium-sized bowl. (Don't worry about the broccoli being slightly warm; it will just bring out the flavors of the chicken and seasonings.) In a separate bowl, mix the marinara, oregano, basil, and salt and pepper to taste, and pour over salad. Top with pepperoni slices and Parmesan cheese.

QUICK TIP

Take this salad to go: The night before, put the raw veggies in a plastic container. Then, instead of cooking broccoli, top the salad with frozen cooked broccoli (it will thaw by lunch tomorrow). Put the chicken and pepperoni slices in a separate baggie, and the marinara mixture in another container. Mix all together just before you eat. If you don't have marinara on hand, it's equally delicious with Italian dressing.

VEG replace chicken with Quorn Naked Chik'n Cutlet; omit pepperoni

VGN omit cheese and pepperoni; replace chicken with Quorn Naked Chik'n Cutlet

D omit cheese; add 1 Tbsp. chopped walnuts

G yes

S yes

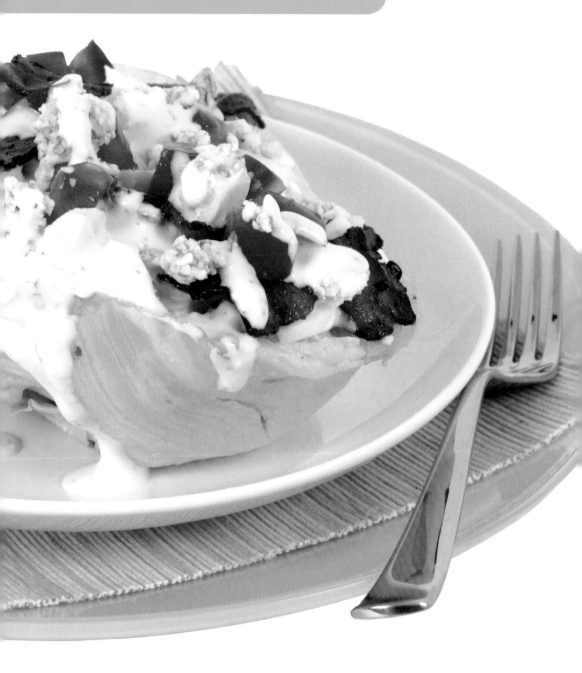

classic wedge salad

0 SUGAR CALORIES, not 430 calories

½ head iceberg lettuce, cut into 2 wedges

2 strips bacon

1 egg

2 Tbsp. diced tomatoes

2 Tbsp. blue cheese, crumbled

2 Tbsp. blue cheese dressing (no sugar added)

Put the egg in a small saucepan, cover with cold water, and bring to a boil. Once at a full rolling boil, cover and turn off the heat. Let stand for 10 to 12 minutes, then drain and cover the egg with cold water to stop the cooking. Let cool, then peel and chop for salad.

Heat a cast-iron skillet and cook the bacon according to package directions. While bacon is cooking, prepare salad in a bowl or on a plate. Lay down the lettuce first, then top with tomatoes, blue cheese crumbles, and chopped egg; drizzle with dressing. After letting the cooked bacon drain on paper towels, crumble over the top and serve.

QUICK TIP

Make hard-boiled eggs early so you have the already-cooled egg ready to go. Consider boiling several eggs at once so you have extra hard-boiled eggs for snacks or other meals.

VEG replace bacon with Lightlife Smart Bacon

VGN replace bacon with Lightlife Smart Bacon, omit egg, omit cheese, use Follow Your Heart Organic Thick & Chunky Bleu Cheese Salad Dressing

D omit cheese, and use Follow Your Heart Organic Thick & Chunky Bleu Cheese Salad Dressing

G use Follow Your Heart Organic Thick & Chunky Bleu Cheese Salad Dressing

S yes

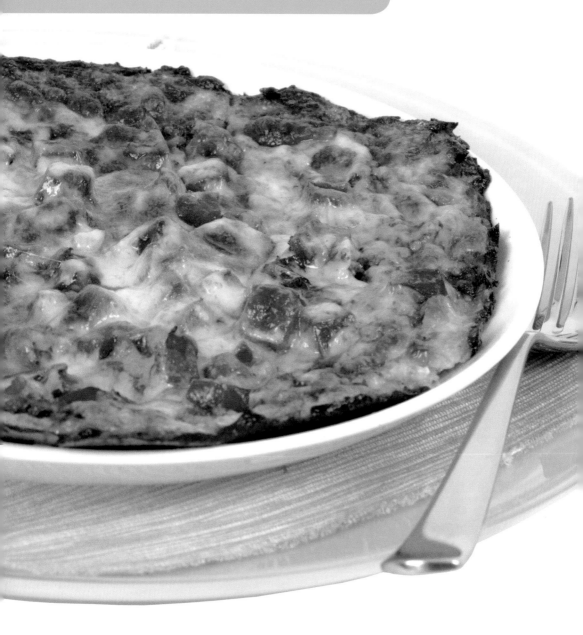

basil pesto pizza

0 SUGAR CALORIES, not 549 calories

½ head cauliflower

¾ cup mozzarella

I egg, lightly beaten

½ tsp. dried oregano

¼ tsp. garlic, minced or pressed

½ tsp. garlic salt

Extra-virgin olive oil

¼ cup pesto

I sliced tomato

I Tbsp. fresh basil, chopped

Salt and pepper

QUICK TIP

Add some extra veggies. Chop up some baby spinach, dice a quarter cup of tomatoes or red bell peppers, and sprinkle them on with the cheese. Or you can make this a salad pizza and top the pie with baby arugula and diced tomatoes just before you eat—add a drizzle of Italian dressing for extra flavor.

Preheat oven to 450°F.

Remove stems and leaves from the cauliflower, and chop into small pieces. Place chopped cauliflower in a food processor, pulse until grain-like, then transfer to a microwave-safe bowl. Microwave on high for about 8 minutes. When done, mix in half of the beaten egg (discard the other half, or reserve and add to your breakfast tomorrow), ½ cup of mozzarella, oregano, garlic, and garlic salt. Transfer the mixture to a cookie sheet sprayed with nonstick cooking spray, and form into a 4"–5" pizza-crust-like round. Brush with olive oil, and bake in center of oven for 15 minutes. When done, top with pesto, tomato, basil, remaining mozzarella, and sprinkle with salt and pepper. Place back in oven for 3 or 4 minutes, until cheese melts.

VEG yes

VGN replace cheese with Daiya Mozzarella Style Shreds, replace egg with Ener-G Egg Replacer, replace pesto with Follow Your Heart Pesto Vegenaise Gourmet

D replace cheese with Daiya Mozzarella Style Shreds, replace pesto with Follow Your Heart Pesto Vegenaise Gourmet

G replace pesto with Follow Your Heart Pesto Vegenaise Gourmet

S yes

turkey caesar salad

0 SUGAR CALORIES, not 220 calories

1 cup romaine lettuce, shredded

¼ cup deli turkey, shredded

1 Tbsp. Parmesan cheese

2 Tbsp. Caesar dressing

Salt and pepper

Put the lettuce in a bowl; top with turkey, Parmesan, dressing, and salt and pepper to taste.

QUICK TIP

Play with your greens.
Mix in a variety of greens such
as baby arugula and spinach
for added texture, flavor,
and nutrients.

VEG replace chicken with Quorn Naked Chik'n Cutlet

VGN omit cheese, replace Caesar dressing with Annie's Naturals Goddess dressing, replace chicken with Quorn Naked Chik'n Cutlet, add 1 Tbsp. chopped walnuts

D replace cheese with 1 Tbsp. chopped walnuts

G yes (but be cautious about the brand of deli meat and dressing; try Boar's Head deli meats and Annie's Naturals Caesar dressing)

S yes (make sure the dressing does not contain anchovies)

dijon salmon

0 SUGAR CALORIES, not 180 calories

1 salmon fillet
1 Tbsp. Dijon mustard
Olive oil
3 asparagus spears, white stems trimmed
½ cup spinach, chopped
Red wine vinegar
Salt and pepper

Turn broiler or grill to high. Brush salmon with olive oil and mustard, and season with salt and pepper. Place in broiler pan or on grill with skin side down, and cook until flaky throughout, about 8–10 minutes. Heat a small nonstick skillet on medium-high, drizzle about ½ tablespoon of olive oil. Add asparagus, season with salt and pepper, and stir frequently until softened. Remove to a plate, arrange spinach alongside, drizzle with more oil and vinegar, then season with salt and pepper and serve with salmon.

QUICK TIP

If asparagus aren't in season, sauté up some sliced zucchini.

VEG choose another option

VGN choose another option

D yes

G yes

S use chicken breast instead of salmon

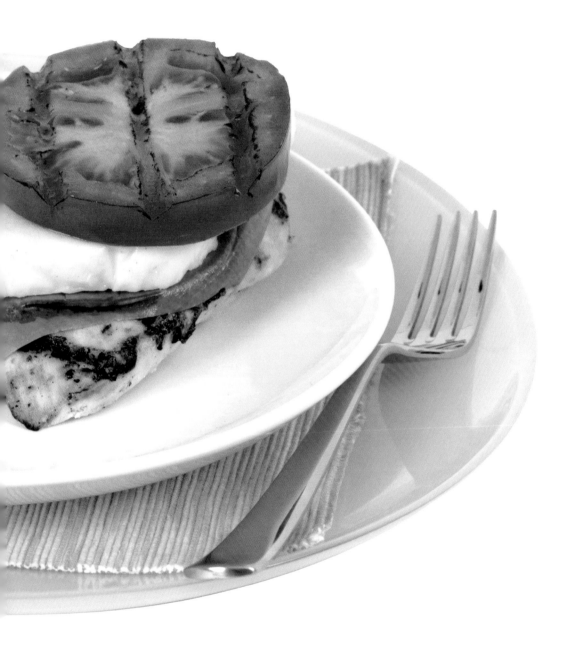

chicken caprese stacks

0 SUGAR CALORIES, not 232 calories

1 chicken breast, skinless and boneless

1 slice fresh mozzarella

2–3 basil leaves

1 slice of tomato

1 Tbsp. olive oil

2 Tbsp. balsamic vinegar

Salt and pepper

Heat the broiler or the grill to high. Brush the chicken with olive oil, and season with salt and pepper on both sides. Broil or grill for 6–8 minutes on each side—if using the broiler, put chicken about 4" below the heat. (Chicken is done when no longer pink and juices run clear, or 165°F in the center with a meat thermometer.) Top the chicken with the basil leaves and slice of mozzarella, and grill or broil for a minute or so, just until cheese begins to melt. You can grill or broil the slice of tomato for a minute or so on each side as well. Then top chicken with tomato, place on a plate, and drizzle with vinegar. Adjust seasoning with salt and pepper.

QUICK TIP

This dish is equally delicious made with turkey-burger patties in place of the chicken breast. Or if you want to bulk up the stack, you can add some grilled, sliced eggplant and peppers.

VEG replace chicken with Quorn Naked Chik'n Cutlet

VGN replace chicken with Quorn Naked Chik'n Cutlet, replace cheese with Tofutti Mozzarella Soy Cheese

D replace cheese with Tofutti Mozzarella Soy Cheese

G yes

S yes

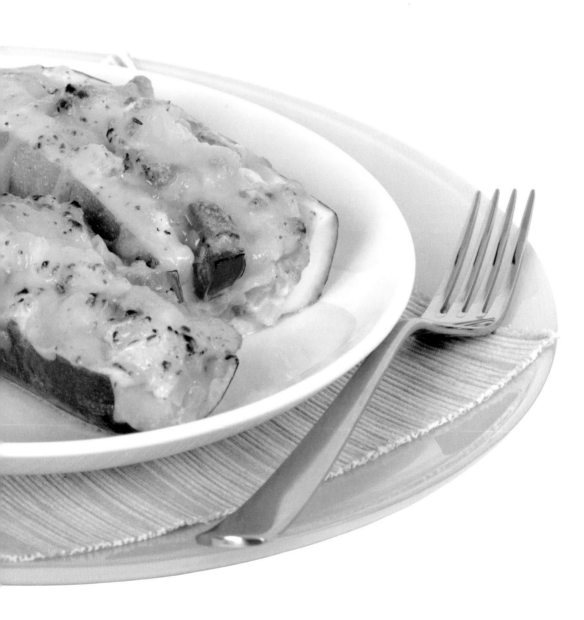

zucchini boats
0 SUGAR CALORIES, not 252 calories

½ zucchini (sliced lengthwise; reserve other half for another use)
1 slice bacon
½ onion, chopped
½ tomato, chopped
1 Tbsp. sour cream
Pinch dried thyme
Pinch curry powder
2 Tbsp. cheddar cheese, shredded
Salt and pepper

Preheat oven to 400°F. Cook bacon in nonstick skillet according to package directions, and drain on paper towels, reserving the bacon grease in the pan. On medium-high heat, add the onion and sauté, stirring frequently for about 5 minutes, until soft. Remove from heat. In a small bowl, crumble the bacon and mix in the tomato and onion. Sprinkle with thyme, and curry, and salt and pepper to taste. Use a spoon to scoop out the seeds in your zucchini half, then fill with the bacon and veggie mixture, and sprinkle cheese on top. Put in an ovenproof dish and bake for 20 minutes, or until cheese starts to bubble and brown.

QUICK TIP

Make it an entrée salad by serving the hot boats on top of a bed of spinach. I like to use a fork and knife to cut and mix them all together. The warm veggies and cheese slightly wilt the spinach, and make a super yummy warm salad. (Many entrées can be transformed into salads this way!)

VEG replace bacon with Lightlife Smart Bacon

VGN replace bacon with Lightlife Smart Bacon; replace sour cream with Follow Your Heart Vegan Gourmet Sour Cream; replace cheese with Daiya Cheddar Style Shreds

D replace sour cream with Follow Your Heart Vegan Gourmet Sour Cream; replace cheese with Daiya Cheddar Style Shreds

G use Boar's Head Bacon

S yes

steak kebab

0 SUGAR CALORIES, not 240 calories

3 oz. steak, cut into 3 chunks

1 thick slice of red onion, cut into 3 pieces

2 chunks of red bell pepper

Olive oil

Salt and pepper

Heat grill on high. Put steak and vegetables in a bowl, drizzle with olive oil, and season with salt and pepper. Skewer the meat and vegetables. Cook, turning often, until meat is cooked through, about 6–8 minutes.

QUICK TIP

You can also add chunks of zucchini, tomatoes, and eggplant to the kebabs. Serve on top of a bed of spinach for extra greens.

VEG add more veggies as desired, or choose another meal

VGN add more veggies as desired, or choose another meal

D yes

G yes

S yes

green greek salad

0 SUGAR CALORIES, not 370 calories

1 chicken breast

2 cups arugula

½ cucumber, chopped

5 cherry tomatoes, halved

5 Kalamata olives, pitted and halved

2 Tbsp. red onion, chopped

1 Tbsp. feta cheese

½ garlic cloves, minced

1 Tbsp. olive oil

1 tsp. lemon juice

½ tsp. red wine vinegar

Salt and pepper

Heat grill or broiler on high. Brush chicken with olive oil, and season with salt and pepper. Place chicken in broiler or on grill and cook until no longer pink inside and juices run clear, about 10 minutes each side. When done, slice chicken thinly.

In a bowl or on a plate, arrange the arugula and top with the chicken, cucumber, tomatoes, olives, onion, and feta cheese. In a bowl, whisk the garlic, olive oil, lemon juice, and vinegar, and drizzle over the salad; season with salt and pepper.

QUICK TIP

If you're taking this dish to work, store the dressing in a separate container and add just before eating so your greens don't get soggy.

VEG replace chicken with Beyond Meat Chicken-Free Strips

VGN omit cheese and substitute 1 Tbsp. of chopped walnuts; replace chicken with Beyond Meat Chicken-Free Strips

D omit cheese and substitute 1 Tbsp. of chopped walnuts

G yes

S yes

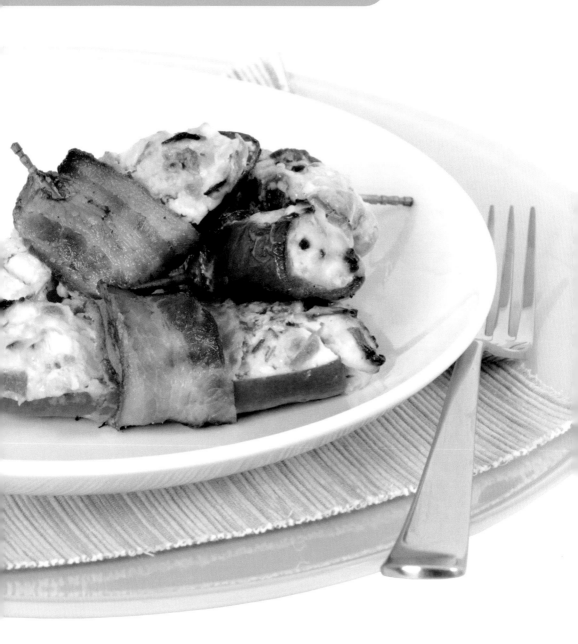

jalapeño bites

0 SUGAR CALORIES, not 347 calories

2 jalapeño peppers, sliced in half lengthwise

1 Tbsp. creamy goat cheese

1 Tbsp. cream cheese

1 Tbsp. Parmesan, grated

1 Tbsp. tomato, chopped

½ Tbsp. fresh cilantro, chopped

4 slices bacon

4 toothpicks

Preheat oven to 375°F. In a bowl, mix together the goat cheese, cream cheese, Parmesan cheese, tomato, and cilantro. Fill the jalapeños with the cheese mixture. Wrap each stuffed jalapeño with 1 slice of bacon and secure it with a toothpick. Place stuffed and wrapped jalapeños in a small baking dish, and put in the middle of the oven for 20 minutes or until bacon is crispy.

QUICK TIP

If you'd like a bit more protein, scramble up an egg to have on the side.

VEG   replace bacon with Lightlife Smart Bacon

VGN   replace cheeses with mashed avocado, replace bacon with Lightlife Smart Bacon

D   replace cheeses with mashed avocado

G   use Boar's Head Bacon

S   yes

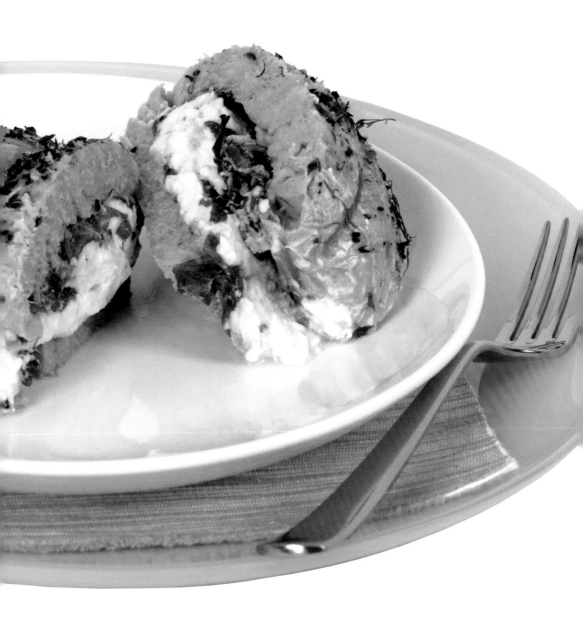

stuffed salmon

0 SUGAR CALORIES, not 231 calories

1 salmon fillet (3–4 oz.)

½ cup spinach, chopped

1 Tbsp. feta cheese

1 Tbsp. ricotta cheese

Olive oil

1 tsp. fresh dill, chopped

1 tsp. dried oregano

Nonstick cooking spray

Salt and pepper

Preheat the oven to 450°F. In a bowl mix together the spinach, feta cheese, and ricotta; season with salt and pepper. With a sharp knife, make a slit into the middle of the salmon and fill with the cheese and vegetable mixture. Brush the stuffed salmon with olive oil, sprinkle on the dill and oregano, and season with salt and pepper. Spray a baking sheet before putting down the fish, then bake for 20 minutes in the center of the oven, or until fish is flaky.

QUICK TIP

Double the recipe and make an extra fillet. Then, for a fast and yummy lunch, serve it chilled on top of a bed of spinach. Add a squeeze of lemon juice and a drizzle of olive oil for a quick dressing.

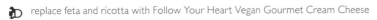

VEG   replace salmon with Quorn Naked Chik'n Cutlet

VGN   replace salmon with Quorn Naked Chik'n Cutlet; replace feta and ricotta with Follow Your Heart Vegan Gourmet Cream Cheese

D   replace feta and ricotta with Follow Your Heart Vegan Gourmet Cream Cheese

G   yes

S   replace salmon with grilled chicken breast

Note: Feel free to add coffee with half-and-half to any breakfast choice.

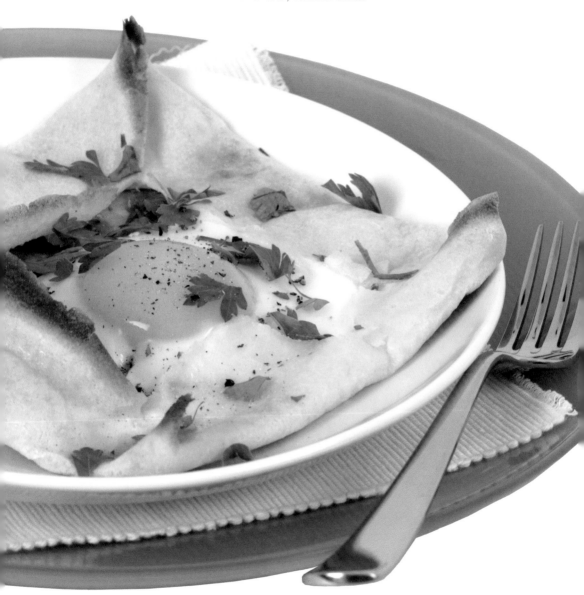

ham and egg crepe square

48 SUGAR CALORIES, not 332 calories

2 Tbsp. flour

1 tsp. Truvia, or 1 Truvia packet

3 Tbsp. half-and-half

½ Tbsp. butter, melted

Canola oil

2 eggs

1 Tbsp. parsley, chopped

1 slice ham, diced

Salt and pepper

Slightly beat one of the eggs, then pour half of it into a small bowl with the flour, and whisk together. Gradually add in the half-and-half until combined. Next, whisk in the butter and a pinch of salt; beat until smooth. Heat a lightly oiled frying pan over medium-high heat. Pour or scoop the batter onto the griddle, making one crepe. Tilt the pan in a circular motion so that the batter coats the surface evenly. Cook the crepe for about 2 minutes, until the bottom is light brown. Loosen with a spatula, turn, and cook the other side. Remove from heat and place on a plate.

Scramble the reserved half egg lightly in the frying pan with the parsley, ham, and salt and pepper; then put it in the crepe. Fry the second egg in the pan, then put it in the crepe and fold the edges into a square shape.

VEG omit ham

VGN choose another option

D omit crepe

G omit flour and use Bob's Red Mill Almond Meal/Flour

S yes

QUICK TIP

For a faster take on this meal, skip the crepe and make this an open-faced ham and egg sandwich. Just scramble both eggs with the ham and seasonings, and serve on top of toasted sourdough or whole-grain bread.

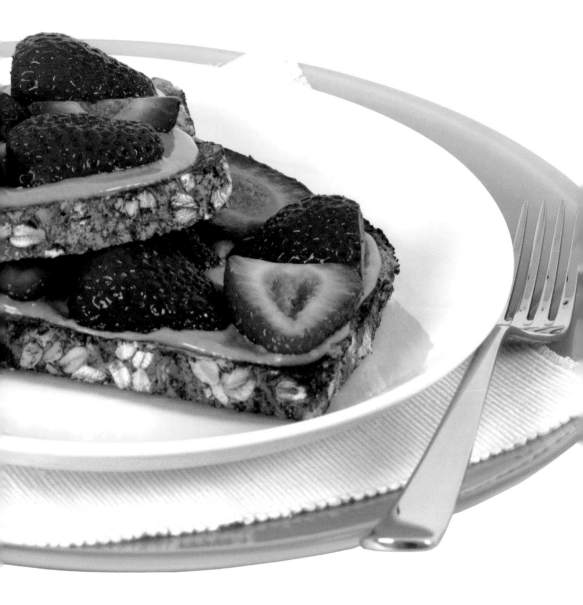

peanut butter and strawberry toasts

144 SUGAR CALORIES, not 350 calories

2 slices whole-grain bread, toasted
1 Tbsp. peanut butter (no sugar added)
¼ cup strawberries, sliced

Spread toast with peanut butter, and top with strawberry slices.

QUICK TIP

You can also top your toast
with ¼ cup sliced bananas
or 1 Tbsp. sugar-free
fruit spread.

VEG   yes

VGN   yes

D   yes

G   use Udi's Gluten-Free Whole-Grain Bread

S   yes

tasty toast

127 SUGAR CALORIES, not 230 calories

2 slices whole-wheat bread, toasted
2 Tbsp. cream cheese
1 Tbsp. sugar-free fruit spread

Spread the cream cheese on top of the toast, and top the cheese with the spread.

QUICK TIP

Add some serotonin-boosting ingredients by topping this toast with ¼ cup sliced strawberries, blueberries, or bananas.

VEG yes

VGN use Tofutti Better Than Cream Cheese instead of cream cheese

D yes

G use Udi's Gluten-Free Whole-Grain Bread

S yes

baja toast

126 SUGAR CALORIES, not 401 calories

2 slices whole-grain bread, toasted
½ avocado, mashed
1 egg, fried
Salt and pepper

Spread toasted bread with mashed avocado and sprinkle with salt and pepper. Top toast with fried egg.

QUICK TIP

Want some extra protein? Top with a couple slices of bacon, sausage, or a small slice of grilled ham.

VEG yes

VGN omit egg, substitute mashed firm tofu sautéed with ¼ tsp. turmeric

D yes

G use Udi's Gluten-Free Whole-Grain Bread

S yes

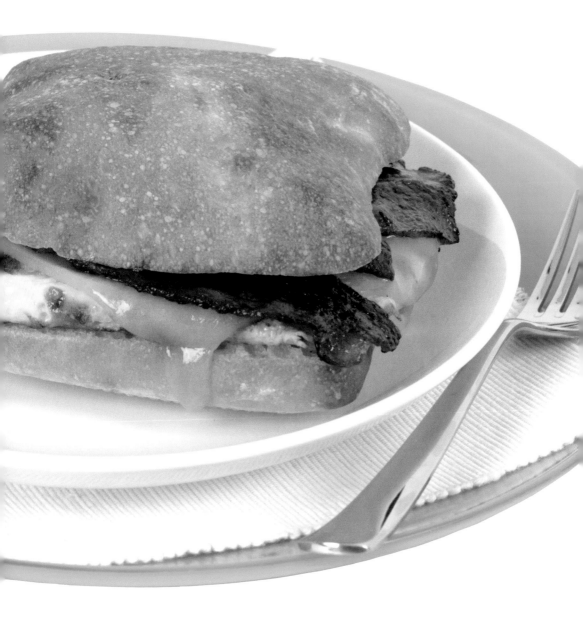

maple bacon sandwich

80 SUGAR CALORIES, not 540 calories

3 slices maple bacon

2 slices cheddar cheese

2 eggs

1 small artisan roll

Butter

Salt and pepper

Heat a cast-iron or nonstick skillet and cook bacon according to package directions. When crisp, remove bacon and drain on paper towels. Turn the skillet heat to low and reserve a small amount of bacon grease.

Beat eggs lightly in a small bowl; turn skillet to high. Add eggs, sprinkled with salt and pepper, then scramble to your liking. When almost done, place the cheese on top of the eggs, turn off the stove, and cover the pan so the cheese melts. Toast and butter the bread, then top with eggs, melted cheese, and bacon. Add salt and pepper to taste.

QUICK TIP

It's a wrap. Heat a whole-wheat tortilla in place of the toast, and make this into a yummy breakfast burrito to eat on-the-go.

VEG replace bacon with Lightlife Smart Bacon

VGN replace bacon with Lightlife Smart Bacon; replace cheese with Daiya Cheddar Style Shreds; omit butter and use Earth Balance Original Buttery Spread or olive oil; omit eggs or substitute mashed firm tofu sautéed with ¼ tsp. turmeric

D replace cheese with Daiya Cheddar Style Shreds; omit butter and use Earth Balance Original Buttery Spread or olive oil

G use Boar's Head Bacon; use Udi's Gluten-Free Whole Grain Bread

S yes

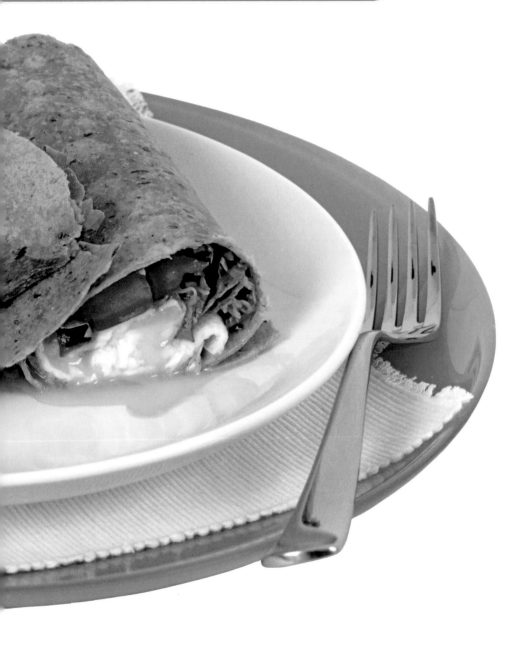

sunshine wrap

42 SUGAR CALORIES, not 163 calories

1 spinach wrap

¼ cup arugula

¼ cup alfalfa sprouts

3 tomato slices

2 eggs

Olive oil or butter

Salt and pepper

Parmesan cheese (optional)

Heat a cast-iron or nonstick skillet, and add a small amount of olive oil or butter. Fry eggs to your liking (over hard works best for a not-so-messy wrap). Heat the wrap for 30 seconds in the microwave, and then fill with eggs, arugula, sprouts, tomato, and salt and pepper. Add a sprinkle of Parmesan if you like, then roll and eat.

VEG yes

VGN omit eggs or substitute mashed firm tofu sautéed with ¼ tsp. turmeric

D omit butter and Parmesan

G use La Tortilla Factory Smart & Delicious Gluten-Free Wraps

S yes

QUICK TIP

Bulk it up. Turn this wrap into a morning salad by increasing the arugula to 1 cup and adding another cup of chopped spinach. Put the veggies in a bowl, and top with eggs—I like mine over medium. Toast a piece of sourdough, butter it, then dice and sprinkle it on top of your salad. Add a drizzle of dressing. The warm eggs bring out the flavors in the salad.

chicks on a nest

120 SUGAR CALORIES, not 390 calories

2 eggs, poached
1 or 2 tsp. vinegar
½ cup spinach
2 slices whole-grain bread, toasted
Butter
Salt and pepper

Fill a small shallow saucepan with about 2" water, and heat to almost boiling; then add 1 or 2 tsp. vinegar (vinegar will help the egg whites congeal). Crack one of the eggs into a small cup, then place the cup near the edge of the hot water and gently pour into water; repeat with the other egg. You can use a spoon to help push the whites closer to the yolks—it helps hold them together. Turn off the heat, cover the pan, and let sit for 4 minutes, until egg whites are cooked.

During the 4-minute sit time, toast and butter the bread, arrange the spinach on a small plate, and sprinkle with salt and pepper. Remove the eggs with a slotted spoon and place on top of the spinach "nest." Serve with the toast.

QUICK TIP

One trick to make the eggs stay somewhat contained is to take a ring from a Mason jar and place it in the pan. Drop the egg over the Mason-jar ring and let it settle, then turn off the heat and cover.

VEG yes

VGN choose another option

D omit butter and use Earth Balance Original Buttery Spread or olive oil

G use Udi's Gluten-Free Whole Grain Bread

S yes

kale and goat cheese scramble

60 SUGAR CALORIES, not 326 calories

2 eggs, lightly beaten

Olive oil or butter

½ garlic clove, minced

1 cup kale leaves, chopped

½ cup water

2 Tbsp. goat cheese, crumbled

1 slice whole-grain bread, toasted

Salt and pepper

Heat a cast-iron or nonstick skillet and heat oil or butter. On medium heat, add garlic and sauté, stirring frequently for one minute, then turn heat to high and add kale and ½ cup water. Cover and cook for 3 minutes. Remove lid and stir until water is almost completely evaporated. Season with salt and pepper, and remove to a bowl. In the same skillet (you may need to wipe it out with a paper towel), add a bit more oil or butter; then add the eggs, scramble until mostly done, and stir in kale. Just before removing the eggs, sprinkle on the cheese. Serve with toasted bread with olive oil or butter.

QUICK TIP

You can also use chopped spinach or mustard greens in place of the kale, and feta cheese in place of the goat cheese.

VEG   yes

VGN   replace cheese with Daiya Cheddar Style Shreds; omit eggs or substitute mashed firm tofu sautéed with ¼ tsp. turmeric

D   replace cheese with Daiya Cheddar Style Shreds

G   use Udi's Gluten-Free Whole Grain Bread

S   yes

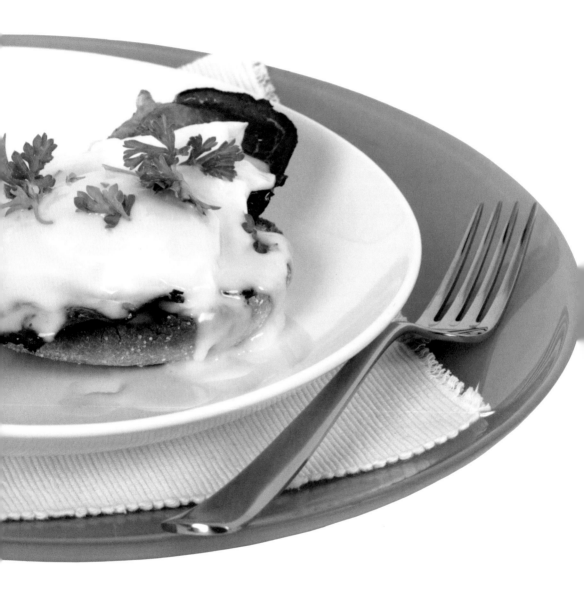

bacon eggs benedict
50 SUGAR CALORIES, not 513 calories

½ English muffin, toasted

Butter

1 or 2 slices of bacon

1 egg

Hollandaise sauce (recipe is below)*

Pinch fresh parsley, chopped

Salt and pepper

QUICK TIP

Feel free to use the more traditional Canadian bacon in place of the regular bacon for the Benedict. I also like to add a slice of tomato to the top of mine.

Heat a cast-iron or nonstick skillet on high. Cook bacon according to package directions, then remove to paper towel to drain. Reserve a bit of the grease and turn down the heat to medium. Add egg and fry to your liking, season with salt and pepper. To serve, butter the English-muffin half and put on a plate, then top with bacon, fried egg, Hollandaise sauce, and parsley. Adjust seasoning with salt and pepper.

*HOLLANDAISE SAUCE RECIPE:

10 Tbsp. butter

3 egg yolks

1 Tbsp. lemon juice

Dash of hot sauce

Salt, to taste

Heat butter in a saucepan until melted. Place egg yolks, lemon juice, hot sauce, and salt in a blender, and blend for 30 seconds on medium speed. Add melted butter and blend on low speed until all butter is combined. Keep warm until served.

(This makes more than 1 serving; save extra for a second breakfast.)

VEG   replace bacon with Lightlife Smart Bacon

VGN choose another option

D   omit Hollandaise sauce and replace butter with Earth Balance Natural Buttery Spread

G   use Food for Life Gluten Free English Muffins

S   yes

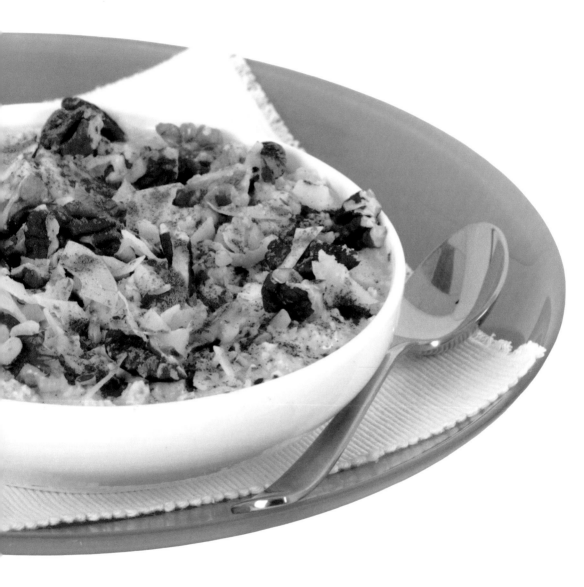

nutty oatmeal

120 SUGAR CALORIES, not 475 calories

¼ cup steel-cut oats

½ tsp. cinnamon

2 Tbsp. unsweetened coconut flakes

1 Tbsp. walnuts, chopped

1 Tbsp. pecans, chopped

¼ cup unsweetened vanilla almond milk

Cook steel-cut oats according to package directions. To serve, place in bowl and sprinkle on coconut, walnuts and pecans. Add almond milk on top.

QUICK TIP

For variety, substitute barley or other unsweetened cooked-cereal grains for the oatmeal.

VEG yes

VGN yes

D yes

G use Bob's Red Mill Gluten Free Steel Cut Oats

S yes

ricotta omelet

104 SUGAR CALORIES, not 385 calories

2 eggs

Olive oil or butter

¼ cup arugula

2 Tbsp. ricotta cheese

1 English muffin, toasted

1 cup spinach

Salt and pepper

For the omelet: Put the eggs in a small bowl and whisk until blended, and season with salt and pepper. Heat a small nonstick skillet on medium low, add about a teaspoon of olive oil or butter, then add the eggs. Let the eggs begin to cook for a minute, then use a heat-resistant rubber spatula to begin pushing the egg into the center, allowing the uncooked portion to flow to the sides—your eggs will begin to look like a yellow pancake. When mostly cooked, but still wet on top, use the spatula to turn your eggs over (if you're adventurous you can also flip your eggs using just the pan). Now add the arugula and ricotta down the middle of the egg, and use the spatula to fold in half. Let sit for about 30 seconds, then turn the folded egg over. Slide onto a plate, and serve with buttered English muffin and spinach alongside.

For the spinach: Heat a cast-iron or nonstick skillet on medium-high, and add a drizzle of olive oil. When hot, toss in the spinach, season with salt and pepper, and stir frequently until just wilted, about 1 or 2 minutes.

QUICK TIP

Substitute a whole-wheat tortilla for the English muffin and roll the omelet inside for a quick on-the-go breakfast.

VEG yes

VGN choose another option

D omit ricotta cheese, or replace with Tofutti, Daiya, or another brand of dairy-free cheese

G use Food for Life Gluten Free English Muffins

S yes

fruity yogurt

33 SUGAR CALORIES, not 145 calories

¼ cup plain Greek yogurt

1 tsp. Truvia

2 Tbsp. almond meal or almond flour (see note)

1 Tbsp. blueberries

1 Tbsp. blackberries

In a bowl, mix the Truvia with yogurt. Sprinkle on the almonds, blueberries, and blackberries.

Note: If you can't find almond flour or meal, just top with chopped almonds, or grind the nuts in a coffee grinder or food processor.

QUICK TIP

This is equally good with sliced strawberries and chopped walnuts.

VEG yes

VGN use WholeSoy & Co Unsweetened Plain Yogurt

D use WholeSoy & Co Unsweetened Plain Yogurt

G yes

S yes

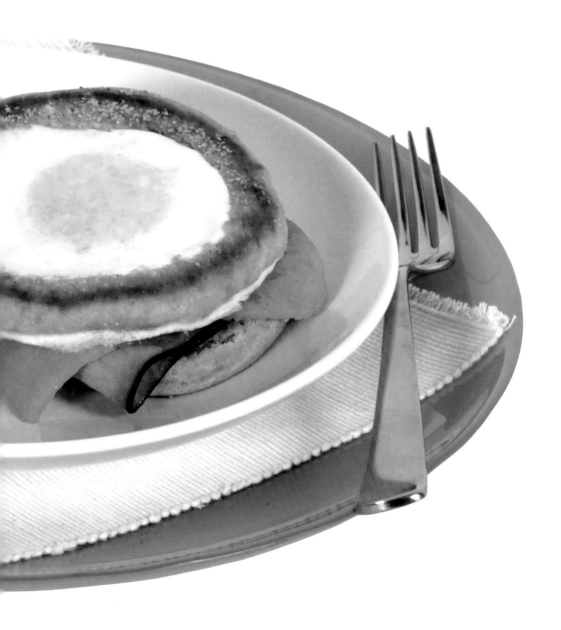

egg-in-a-hole sandwich

53 SUGAR CALORIES, not 282 calories

1 egg
Butter or olive oil
1 slice Canadian bacon
½ whole-wheat English muffin
1 slice cheddar cheese
Salt and pepper

Press down on English muffin with a glass to create a hole in the muffin's center. Heat a cast-iron or nonstick skillet on medium-high and heat butter or olive oil, then add both the muffin with the hole and the muffin center to the pan (make sure the side with the nooks and crannies faces down). Add Canadian bacon to pan. Crack the egg into the hole in the middle of the muffin, season with salt and pepper, and cook till whites look done to your liking. Then carefully flip over the muffin with the egg, the muffin center, and the bacon. Remove muffin center to a plate, then top with the bacon, cheese, then the muffin with egg. Cover the stack with an inverted glass bowl for a minute to help the cheese melt.

QUICK TIP

You can use a slice of toast in place of the muffin.

VEG   replace bacon with Yves Meatless Canadian Bacon

VGN   choose another option

D   replace cheese with Tofutti American Soy-Cheese Slices

G   use Food for Life Gluten Free English Muffins, use Hormel Canadian Bacon

S   yes

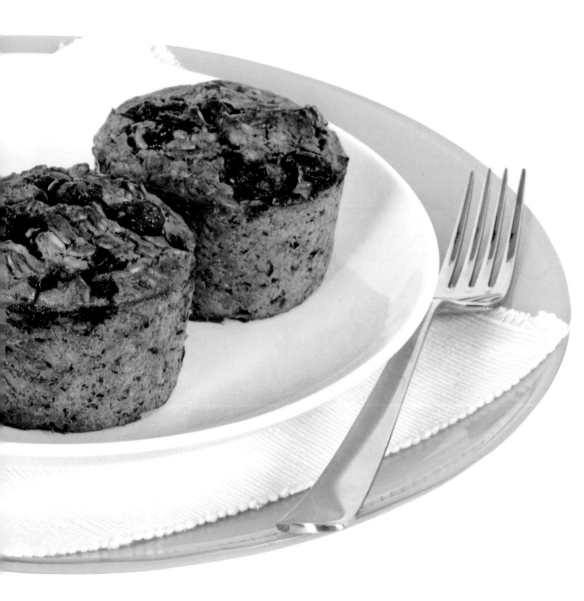

baked oatmeal muffins

78 SUGAR CALORIES, not 144 calories

(SERVING SIZE: 2 MUFFINS)

1 egg

1 tsp. vanilla extract

1⅓ cups unsweetened applesauce

2¾ cups half-and-half

⅔ cup banana, mashed

4 packs stevia

3⅓ cups oats

¼ cup ground flaxseed

1 Tbsp. cinnamon

3 tsp. baking powder

1 tsp. salt

1 cup blueberries

Preheat oven to 350°F, and line a muffin tin with 12 cupcake liners. In a bowl, mix the egg, vanilla, applesauce, half-and-half, and banana. In another bowl, mix the stevia, oats, flaxseed, cinnamon, baking powder, and salt. Mix the dry ingredients into the wet until well blended. Divide the mixture evenly in the 12 muffin cups, and top with a few blueberries each. Bake in the middle of oven for 30 minutes.

QUICK TIP

Leftover muffins can be frozen and heated in the microwave for 45 seconds for an on-the-go breakfast on another morning.

VEG   yes

VGN   replace eggs with Ener-G Egg Replacer; replace half-and-half with unsweetened almond milk

D   replace half-and-half with unsweetened almond milk

G   use Bob's Red Mill Gluten Free Thick Rolled Oats

S   yes

fruit and nut yogurt
8 SUGAR CALORIES, not 211 calories

¼ cup plain Greek yogurt

1 Truvia packet

2 Tbsp. sliced almonds

3 strawberries, sliced

In a bowl, combine the yogurt and the Truvia; mix well. Top with almonds and strawberry slices.

QUICK TIP

This is equally good with other berries such as black-berries or blueberries, and you can swap out the nuts for chopped walnuts or pine nuts.

VEG yes

VGN substitute So Delicious Greek Dairy Free Coconut Milk Plain "Yogurt"

D substitute So Delicious Greek Dairy Free Coconut Milk Plain "Yogurt"

G yes

S yes

ricotta toast

102 SUGAR CALORIES, not 210 calories

2 slices whole-wheat bread, toasted

2 Tbsp. ricotta cheese

2 Tbsp. sugar-free preserves

Spread the toast with ricotta, then top with preserves.

QUICK TIP

No ricotta? Use cottage cheese in its place. You can also top with sliced straw-berries in place of the preserves.

VEG yes

VGN substitute 2 Tbsp. peanut butter in place of ricotta

D substitute 2 Tbsp. peanut butter in place of ricotta

G use Udi's Gluten-Free Whole Grain Bread

S yes

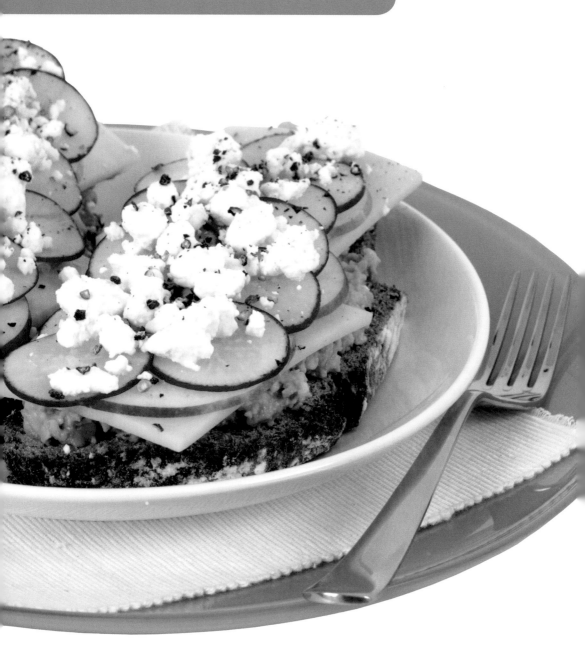

open-faced avocado sandwich

65 SUGAR CALORIES, not 241 calories

1 slice pumpernickel bread, toasted

¼ avocado

1 slice provolone cheese

1 or 2 radishes, sliced thinly

¼ apple, cut into 5 thin slices

2 Tbsp. goat cheese, crumbled

Salt and pepper

Preheat broiler. In a small bowl mash avocado, and add salt and pepper to taste. Spread the toast with avocado; top with radishes, apples, provolone, and goat cheese; and sprinkle with salt and pepper. Place under broiler just until cheese melts, 1 minute.

VEG yes

VGN replace cheeses with Tofutti, Daiya, or another brand of dairy-free cheese

D replace cheeses with Tofutti, Daiya, or another brand of dairy-free cheese

G use Udi's Gluten-Free Whole-Grain Bread

S yes

QUICK TIP

You can easily turn this Happy recipe into a Slim version by creating avocado cups instead of a sandwich—no need for a broiler either. Just dice up the provolone, radishes, and apple, and toss with the goat cheese; salt and pepper to taste. Slice an avocado in half, take out the seed, and fill one of the avocado halves with the mixture, reserving the other half for another meal. Serve on a bed of baby spinach or lettuce. Still want the Happy? Just have a slice of toast on the side.

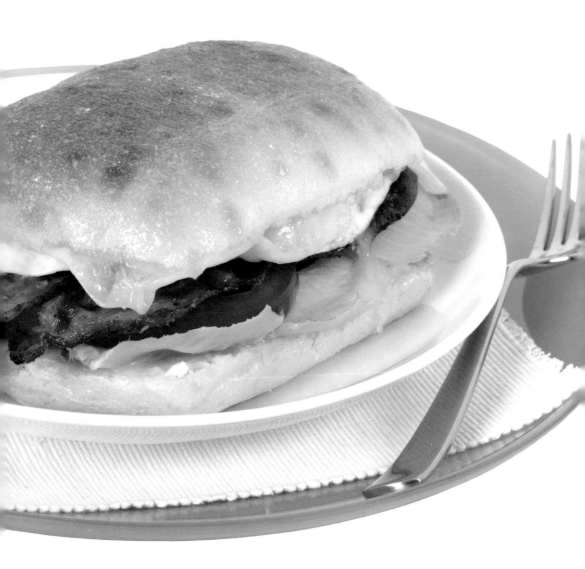

blt egg sandwich
160 SUGAR CALORIES, not 533 calories

1 small artisan roll, toasted
1 Tbsp. mayonnaise
4 slices bacon
Romaine lettuce
3 tomato slices
1 slice pepper Jack cheese (enough to cover the bread)
1 egg
Salt and pepper

Heat a cast-iron or nonstick skillet and cook the bacon according to package directions; drain on paper towels, reserving a tablespoon of bacon grease in the pan. Fry the egg in the same pan to your liking.

Spread the mayo on the toasted bread and add the toppings in any order you like. Top with salt and pepper to taste.

VEG omit bacon

VGN omit bacon and egg; use Tofutti, Daiya, or another brand of dairy-free cheese

D use Tofutti, Daiya, or another brand of cheese alternative

G use Boar's Head bacon and Udi's Gluten-Free Whole Grain Bread

S yes

QUICK TIP

You can always use fresh spinach leaves or arugula in place of lettuce on your sandwich. Remember, the darker the green, the more antioxidants and vitamins it has.

feta pita pizza

67 SUGAR CALORIES, not 248 calories

½ whole-wheat pita bread (sliced so that the round is still whole)

Olive oil

2 Tbsp. Alfredo sauce

Feta cheese, crumbled, to taste

2 Tbsp. black or Greek olives, pitted and sliced

1 Tbsp. red onion, chopped

1 Tbsp. sun-dried tomatoes (the kind packed in oil), drained and chopped

1 Tbsp. chopped fresh basil

Salt and pepper

Preheat oven to 450°F. Brush the pita with a bit of olive oil and spread with Alfredo sauce. Sprinkle on feta, olives, red onion, sun-dried tomatoes, and basil; salt and pepper to taste. Place on nonstick baking sheet and cook for 5 to 7 minutes, or until topping is bubbly and beginning to brown. You can also heat this pizza in a toaster oven. Just watch closely so it doesn't burn.

QUICK TIP

This is a good recipe to have fun with. If you don't care for Alfredo sauce or want something different, you can substitute pesto or marinara sauce (no sugar added) for the spread. For toppings you can add some sliced sautéed onions, zucchini, eggplant, or spinach. No pita? You can use a whole-wheat tor-tilla in its place.

VEG yes

VGN replace feta with Daiya Mozzarella Style Shreds; replace Alfredo with pesto or marinara sauce

D replace feta with Daiya Mozzarella Style Shreds; replace Alfredo with pesto or marinara sauce

G use Udi's Gluten-Free Whole-Grain tortilla

S yes

sweet spinach salad

139 SUGAR CALORIES, not 711 calories

1–2 cups baby spinach, washed

1–2 Tbsp. olive oil

½ lemon

¼ pear, diced

2 Tbsp. pecans, chopped

¼ cup blue cheese, crumbled

Salt and pepper

1 small baguette or whole-wheat bread, toasted

Butter

Put spinach in a medium-sized bowl or on a plate; if the pieces are too big, give them a quick chopping. Drizzle on the olive oil, squeeze on lemon juice, and sprinkle with salt and pepper. Top with the pear, pecans, and blue cheese crumbles. Taste, and add more salt and pepper, if needed. Serve with warm baguette or toast, topped with butter.

QUICK TIP

Get handy—swap out the baguette for a whole-wheat tortilla to turn this salad into an on-the-go wrap. Just put the salad mixture in the tortilla, and roll.

VEG yes

VGN omit butter and use Earth Balance Original Buttery Spread or olive oil; replace cheeses with Tofutti, Daiya, or another brand of dairy-free cheese

D omit butter and use Earth Balance Original Buttery Spread or olive oil; replace cheeses with Tofutti, Daiya, or another brand of dairy-free cheese

G omit the baguette, or use Udi's Gluten-Free Whole-Grain Bread

S yes

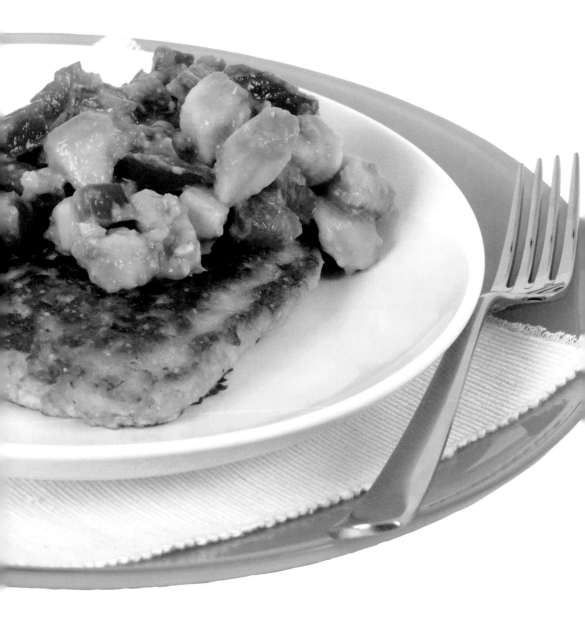

HAPPY DAYS RECIPES

spicy corn cakes

87 SUGAR CALORIES, not 412 calories

½ ear corn, shucked

2 Tbsp. flour

1 Tbsp. cornmeal

½ Tbsp. red onion, diced

½ Tbsp. fresh basil, chopped

Pinch baking powder

Pinch baking soda

1 egg

1 tsp. buttermilk

1 tsp. butter, melted

Olive oil

2 Tbsp. tomato, chopped

2 Tbsp. avocado, diced

Pinch cilantro, chopped

Salt and pepper

Pulse the corn kernels in a food processor or blender, or chop finely by hand. In a bowl, mix the kernels with the flour, cornmeal, red onion, basil, baking powder, baking soda, and a sprinkle of salt and pepper; set aside. In a coffee mug or small bowl, whisk the egg with a fork and measure out approximately ¼ of the egg mixture into another small bowl (reserve the remaining egg to scramble for your breakfast, or toss). Mix the egg with the buttermilk and melted butter, then add to the cornmeal mixture and mix well.

Heat a cast-iron or nonstick skillet, and add a drizzle of olive oil. When the oil is hot, add the batter and cook each side until golden brown and cooked through. Serve topped with the tomato, avocado, and cilantro. Adjust salt and pepper seasoning as needed.

VEG yes

VGN omit egg and use Ener-G Egg Replacer, omit buttermilk and use unsweetened coconut milk, omit butter and use Earth Balance Original Buttery Spread or olive oil

D omit buttermilk and use unsweetened coconut milk; omit butter and use Earth Balance Original Buttery Spread or olive oil

G omit flour and use Bob's Red Mill Almond Meal/Flour

S yes

QUICK TIP

Pump up the protein! If you feel like you want a heartier meal, add a couple slices of bacon or a couple tablespoons of shredded cheddar cheese.

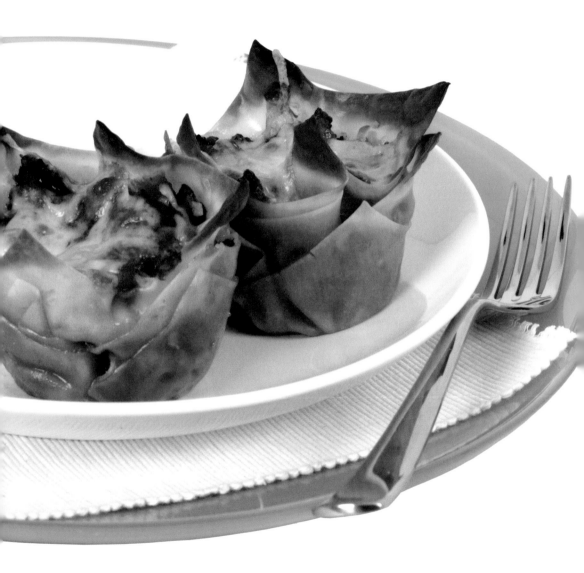

lasagna cups

119 SUGAR CALORIES, not 741 calories

6 wonton wrappers

Parmesan cheese, grated (for topping, add to taste)

Mozzarella, shredded (for topping, add to taste)

½ cup ricotta

¼ cup ground beef, cooked

¼ cup marinara sauce

Salt and pepper

Preheat oven to 375°F. Oil two muffin-tin cups and line with one wonton wrapper each. In a small bowl, mix the cheeses and the ground beef, and season with salt and pepper. Put ⅓ of the mixture in the bottom of the wonton wrappers, and top with a spoonful of marinara sauce; repeat this two more times, then top with more sprinkles of Parmesan and mozzarella. Bake on the center rack in your oven for 20 minutes or until cheese is bubbly.

VEG omit meat and substitute BOCA Ground Crumbles

VGN omit Parmesan; replace mozzarella with Daiya Mozzarella Style Shreds; use crumbled tofu or Tofutti Better than Ricotta Cheese instead of ricotta; omit meat and substitute BOCA Ground Crumbles

D omit Parmesan; replace mozzarella with Daiya Mozzarella Style Shreds; use crumbled tofu or Tofutti Better than Ricotta Cheese instead of ricotta

G omit wonton wrappers

S yes

QUICK TIP

Make ahead for a fast breakfast or lunch; these little cups freeze up wonderfully. Make the recipe as directed and let cool on top of the stove, then wrap each one individually in plastic and freeze. When you are ready to eat, you can just unwrap one and heat it for a minute in the microwave.

zucchini linguine

164 SUGAR CALORIES, not 447 calories

2 oz. linguine

    (Tip: a one-pound box of linguine has eight 2-oz. servings,

    which is about ¾ cup when cooked)

10 slices zucchini

½ garlic clove, minced

¼ cup goat cheese

Olive oil

½ tsp. lemon juice

Salt and pepper

Cook linguine according to package directions. Meanwhile heat a skillet and add a drizzle of olive oil. When hot, add the zucchini slices and garlic, and sauté on medium for about 5 minutes, or until just tender crisp. Remove skillet from heat. After you drain the linguine, add it to the skillet and turn the heat on low. Sprinkle on goat cheese, a bit more olive oil, and the lemon juice, and season with salt and pepper to taste. Heat until the goat cheese starts to warm, just a minute or so.

VEG yes

VGN omit cheese, add 1 Tbsp. chopped walnuts

D omit cheese, add 1 Tbsp. chopped walnuts

G use Lundberg Brown Rice Pasta

S yes

QUICK TIP

Play with your pasta. This is a great recipe for experimentation, depending on your preferences. If you want a bit more protein, add some shredded cooked chicken, diced ham, or chopped nuts. Use quinoa pasta for more fiber and a vegetarian source of protein. For extra nutrients and antioxidants, add some Freebie Foods such as baby spinach, diced red bell peppers, or tomatoes.

catch of the day

35 SUGAR CALORIES, not 226 calories

1 halibut fillet

Olive oil

½ cup broccoli, cut into bite-size pieces

Butter

¼ cup wild rice, cooked

Salt and pepper

The rice: Cook in a rice cooker, or on the stove according to package directions.

The fish: Heat a nonstick skillet on medium-high and add a drizzle of olive oil. Meanwhile, season the fish with salt and pepper on both sides. When the oil is hot, but not smoking, add the fillet and cook for 3 minutes, then turn and cook for another 3 minutes.

The broccoli: Add water to cover the bottom of a pan with a steamer basket. Bring the water to a boil, then reduce the heat to medium, and add broccoli. Cover and let cook for 7 minutes, then remove broccoli while still tender crisp and place in a bowl. Toss with butter, and season with salt and pepper.

QUICK TIP

Swap the fillet. Feel free to use any similar cut of fish in this recipe; it is equally delicious with salmon, sea bass, or tilapia.

VEG   use Sophie's Kitchen Breaded Vegan Fish Fillets in place of halibut

VGN   use Sophie's Kitchen Breaded Vegan Fish Fillets in place of halibut; use more olive oil or Earth Balance Original Buttery Spread instead of butter

D   use more olive oil or Earth Balance Original Buttery Spread instead of butter

G   yes

S   choose another option

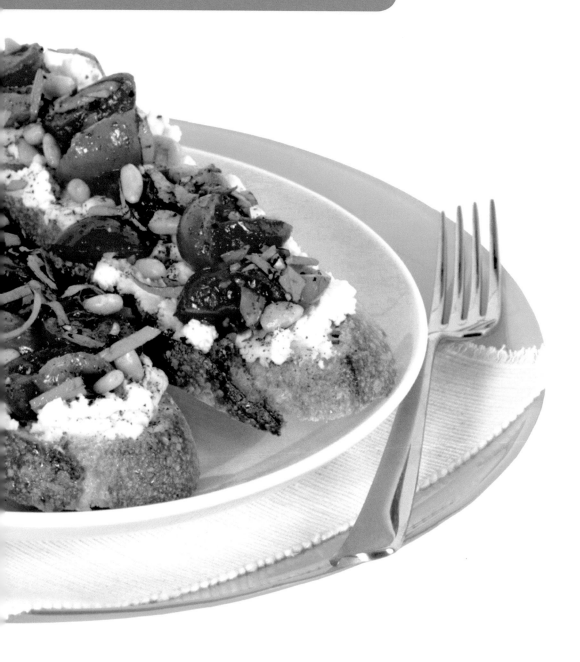

heirloom tomato toasts

160 SUGAR CALORIES, not 650 calories

Olive oil

1 Tbsp. fresh basil, chopped

4 tomato slices (heirloom recommended, but optional)

1 garlic clove, minced

Salt and pepper

2 small slices whole-grain baguette, lightly toasted

3 Tbsp. feta cheese

3 Tbsp. goat cheese

2 Tbsp. pine nuts

Preheat broiler. Heat a small skillet and add a drizzle of olive oil. When hot, add garlic, basil, and tomatoes and sauté for a few minutes, until soft. Season with salt and pepper.

In a small bowl, mix together both cheeses with a fork, then mash and spread onto toasts. Top with pine nuts, and place under broiler for a minute, just until cheese is melted. Top with the tomato mixture.

QUICK TIP

No pine nuts on hand? This recipe is equally good with a sprinkle of chopped walnuts, almonds, or macadamia nuts.

VEG yes

VGN replace cheeses with Follow Your Heart Vegan Gourmet Cream Cheese

D replace cheeses with Follow Your Heart Vegan Gourmet Cream Cheese

G use Schar gluten-free baguette

S yes

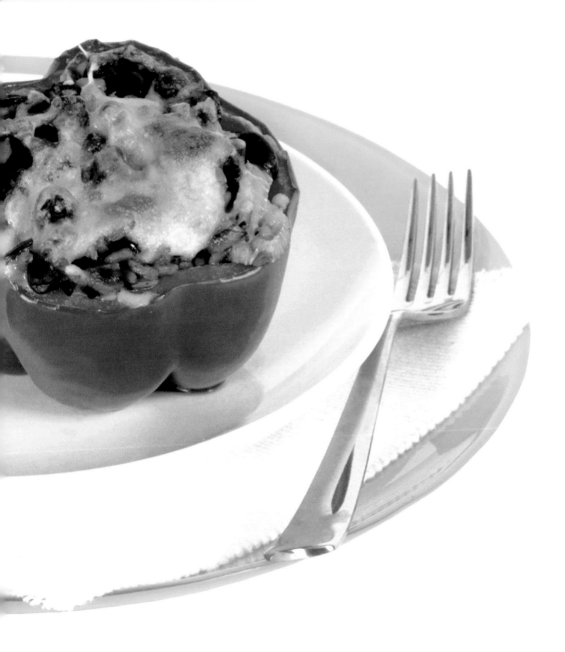

rice and bean stuffed pepper

120 SUGAR CALORIES, not 328 calories

¼ onion, chopped

½ celery stalk, chopped

½ garlic clove, minced

¼ cup spinach, chopped

¼ cup black beans (canned is fine, rinsed and drained)

¼ cup cooked rice

2 Tbsp. pepper Jack cheese, shredded

1 red bell pepper, top and seeds removed

1 tsp. cumin

Olive oil

Salt and pepper

Preheat oven to 350°F.

Heat a cast-iron or nonstick skillet; drizzle with olive oil. Add onion and celery, and sauté on medium-high for 5 minutes, stirring often. Sauté garlic for a minute, then add spinach and continue cooking until just wilted, then remove from heat. In a bowl, mix the veggies, beans, rice, cheese, cumin, and salt and pepper to taste. Fill the bell pepper with the mixture, place in baking dish, cover with aluminum foil, and bake in center of oven for 1 hour.

VEG yes

VGN replace cheese with Daiya Pepperjack Style Shreds

D replace cheese with Daiya Pepperjack Style Shreds

G yes

S yes

QUICK TIP

You can make these peppers the night before, and reheat for lunch or dinner the following day. About 2 minutes in the microwave per pepper.

rockin' ravioli

100 SUGAR CALORIES, not 170 calories

5 whole-wheat cheese ravioli

1 Tbsp. Parmesan cheese, grated

½ cup broccoli, cut into small pieces

Olive oil

Salt and pepper

Cook ravioli according to package directions, and drain. Put a steamer basket in a saucepan with enough water to cover bottom of pan, and bring to a boil. Add broccoli, then cover and steam for 5 minutes, or until broccoli is bright green. Serve ravioli on a bowl or plate, topped with broccoli, a drizzle of olive oil, Parmesan, and salt and pepper to taste.

QUICK TIP

This dish is equally good at room temperature or chilled. Serve on top of a bed of chopped spinach for "pasta salad."

VEG yes

VGN use a whole-wheat pasta in place of the ravioli and replace cheese with Daiya Cheddar Style Shreds

D use a whole-wheat pasta in place of the ravioli, and replace cheese with Daiya Cheddar Style Shreds

G use Lundberg Elbow Brown Rice Pasta or another gluten-free pasta brand

S yes

prosciutto wrap

80 SUGAR CALORIES, not 290 calories

1 whole-wheat wrap

1 Tbsp. pesto

2 Tbsp. goat cheese, crumbled

3 asparagus stalks, white stems trimmed

3 slices prosciutto

Salt and pepper

Heat a cast-iron or nonstick skillet on medium-high, and add a drizzle of olive oil. When hot, add the asparagus; stir often for 10 minutes. Remove and chop the stalks you'll use. Heat wrap in microwave for 30 seconds. Spread on pesto, then add cheese, asparagus, and prosciutto. Season with salt and pepper, roll, and eat.

QUICK TIP

Cook extra asparagus and save them for snacking. Try swapping 3 slices of cooked bacon for the prosciutto. You can also make this an open-faced sandwich by substituting a slice of sourdough toast for the wrap.

VEG omit prosciutto and add 1 Tbsp. chopped walnuts

VGN omit prosciutto and add 1 Tbsp. chopped walnuts; replace goat cheese with Daiya Cheddar Style Shreds

D replace goat cheese with Daiya Cheddar Style Shreds

G use La Tortilla Factory Smart & Delicious Gluten-Free Wraps

S yes

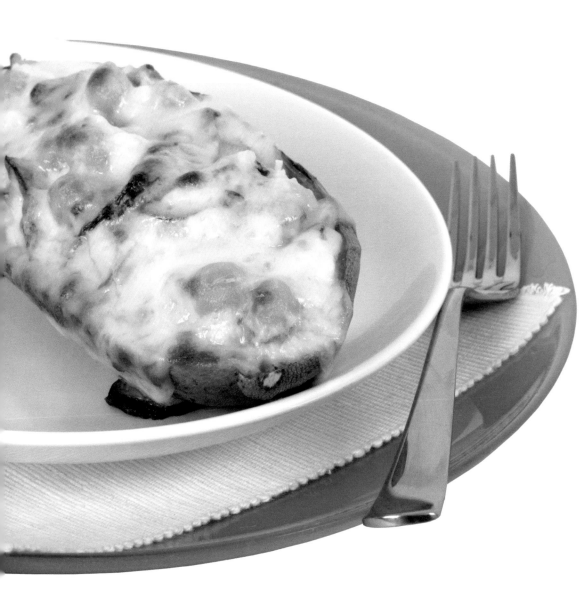

sweet potato skins

79 SUGAR CALORIES, not 206 calories

½ sweet potato (sliced lengthwise; reserve other half for another use)

Olive oil

½ shallot, minced

I cup spinach, chopped

2 Tbsp. chickpeas (canned are fine, rinsed and
drained)

I Tbsp. cream cheese

I Tbsp. sour cream

¼ cup mozzarella

Salt and pepper

QUICK TIP

No time to bake a potato? Turn these skins into an open-faced sandwich by putting the topping on a piece of whole-wheat toast. This is also fantastic with feta or goat cheese sprinkled on top instead of the mozzarella.

Preheat oven 350°F. Wrap sweet potato loosely in foil and place in oven on baking sheet for 45 to 60 minutes. While sweet potato is baking, prepare the vegetables.

Heat a cast-iron or nonstick skillet on medium-high heat, and add a drizzle of olive oil. When oil is hot, sauté the shallot for a couple minutes, then add spinach and cook until just wilted. Season with salt and pepper, and remove from heat. In a bowl, mix together the sautéed vegetables, chickpeas, cream cheese, and sour cream, and adjust salt and pepper if needed.

When sweet potato is done and cool enough to handle, scoop out most of the flesh and discard or save for another use. Fill with cheese/veggie mixture, and return to oven for 5 minutes. Top with mozzarella and bake until cheese is melted, about 3 more minutes.

VEG yes

VGN replace cream cheese with Follow Your Heart Vegan Gourmet Cream Cheese, replace sour cream with Follow Your Heart Gourmet Sour Cream, replace cheese with Tofutti Mozzarella Soy Cheese

D replace cream cheese with Follow Your Heart Vegan Gourmet Cream Cheese, replace sour cream with Follow Your Heart Gourmet Sour Cream, replace cheese with Tofutti Mozzarella Soy Cheese

G yes

S yes

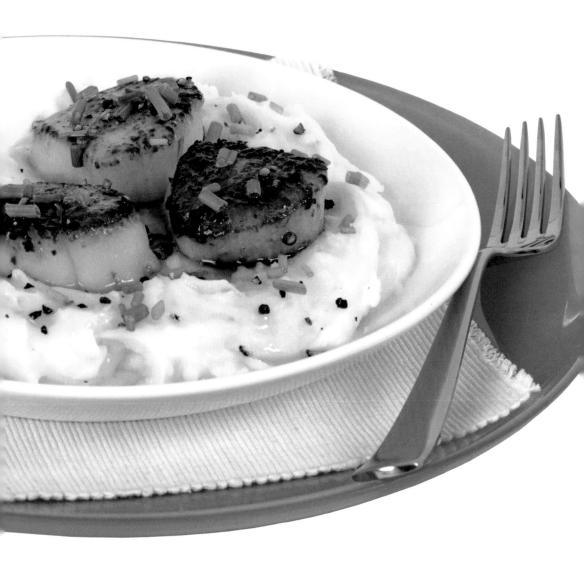

sautéed scallops

72 SUGAR CALORIES, not 480 calories

3–6 scallops

Olive oil

1 potato

2 Tbsp. butter

2 Tbsp. half-and-half

1 Tbsp. fresh chives, chopped

Salt and pepper

QUICK TIP

The scallops are also delicious served on top of ½ cup of cooked brown rice.

To make scallops: Rinse scallops and blot with paper towels so that they are fairly dry. Heat a nonstick skillet on medium low, and add a drizzle of olive oil and 1 tablespoon of the butter. When butter is melted, turn the heat to medium and add the scallops. Cook for 2 minutes, or until brown, then turn and cook for another 2 minutes. Remove, and season with salt and pepper.

To make mashed potatoes: Peel and quarter one potato. Place in a microwave-safe bowl with a lid, and cook on high for 6–8 minutes. Let stand for another 5 minutes with the lid on, then check for tenderness when pierced with a fork. Add the other tablespoon of butter and the half-and-half, then mash with a fork and season with salt and pepper.

To serve: Arrange ½ cup mashed potatoes on a plate. Top with scallops, chopped chives, and more salt and pepper to taste.

VEG replace scallops with sautéed tofu cubes

VGN replace scallops with sautéed tofu cubes; replace butter with Earth Balance Natural Buttery Spread

D replace butter with Earth Balance Natural Buttery Spread

G yes

S replace scallops with grilled chicken strips

penne marinara

156 SUGAR CALORIES, not 300 calories

2 oz. whole-wheat penne pasta

    (Tip: A one-pound box of penne has eight 2-oz. servings, or about ¾ cup, cooked)

1 Italian sausage

2 Tbsp. marinara sauce (no sugar added)

½ garlic clove, minced

Olive oil

1 cup spinach, chopped

Salt and pepper

Parmesan or feta cheese (optional)

Cook pasta and sausage according to package directions. Heat a cast-iron or nonstick skillet on medium-high heat, and add a drizzle of olive oil. When hot, sauté garlic for a minute, then add spinach and stir until just wilted. Season with salt and pepper; then stir in sausage, penne, and marinara. Serve with a sprinkling of Parmesan or feta cheese, if you desire.

VEG omit sausage and use BOCA Ground Crumbles

VGN omit sausage and use BOCA Ground Crumbles, omit cheeses

D omit cheeses

G use Lundberg Brown Rice Pasta

S yes

QUICK TIP

Any type of pasta will work in this recipe, but smaller shapes are better at catching the sauce. For another gluten-free option than the one below, you can make this recipe with cooked brown rice instead of pasta.

savory kebab

90 SUGAR CALORIES, not 255 calories

½ cup brown rice, cooked

3 oz. chicken, cut into kebab-size chunks

½ cup eggplant, cut into 1" chunks

½ red bell pepper, cut into chunks

1 Tbsp. olive oil

2 Tbsp. soy sauce

Pepper

Make rice according to package directions. In a bowl, mix together olive oil, soy sauce, and pepper. Put chicken and vegetables into marinade and refrigerate for 2 hours. Heat grill or broiler to high. Drain marinade and discard, then thread the chicken and vegetables onto a skewer. Put skewer on grill or in broiler, and cook for 12–15 minutes until chicken is cooked. Serve over brown rice.

VEG use cubed seasoned tofu in place of meat

VGN use cubed seasoned tofu in place of meat

D yes

G yes

S yes

QUICK TIP

Bulk up your veggies. Add some onions and quartered tomatoes to the kebabs. You can also mix ½ cup chopped spinach into the hot rice just before serving. The heat of the rice will wilt the spinach perfectly.

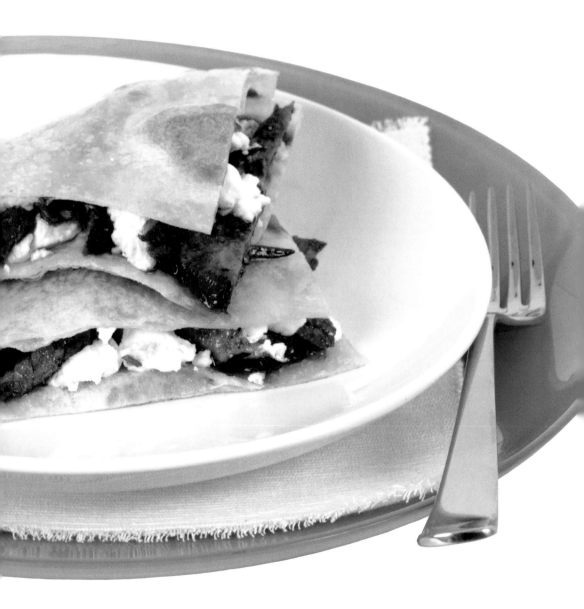

steak and goat cheese quesadilla

127 SUGAR CALORIES, not 455 calories

3 oz. strip or flank steak

Olive oil

5 slices red onion

¼ cup baby spinach leaves, chopped

2 Tbsp. goat cheese, crumbled

1 Tbsp. balsamic vinegar

2 whole-wheat tortillas, 6" diameter

Nonstick cooking spray

Salt and pepper

Rosemary (1 sprig, chopped)

QUICK TIP

You can also serve this dish as a burrito. Heat one large whole-wheat tortilla, fill it with the toppings, then roll.

The steak: Heat your grill or broiler to high, and brush the steak with olive oil and season with salt and pepper. Place on grill or broiler, and cook on each side for 4–5 minutes until done to your liking. Remove from heat and let rest for 5–10 minutes, then slice thinly.

The quesadilla: Heat a cast-iron or nonstick skillet on medium-high, spray with nonstick spray if needed. When hot, add one tortilla and layer on the steak, cheese, onion, rosemary, and spinach, and season with salt and pepper. Top with second tortilla, let sit for a minute or two. When bottom tortilla begins to crisp and brown, use a spatula to carefully turn over and brown the second side. Cut into wedges and drizzle on a bit of the vinegar, or use as a dip.

VEG   replace steak with Lightlife Smart Strips Steak

VGN   replace steak with Lightlife Smart Strips Steak, replace cheese
          with Daiya Pepperjack Style Shreds

D   replace cheese with Daiya Pepperjack Style Shreds

G   use Mission Corn Tortillas

S   yes

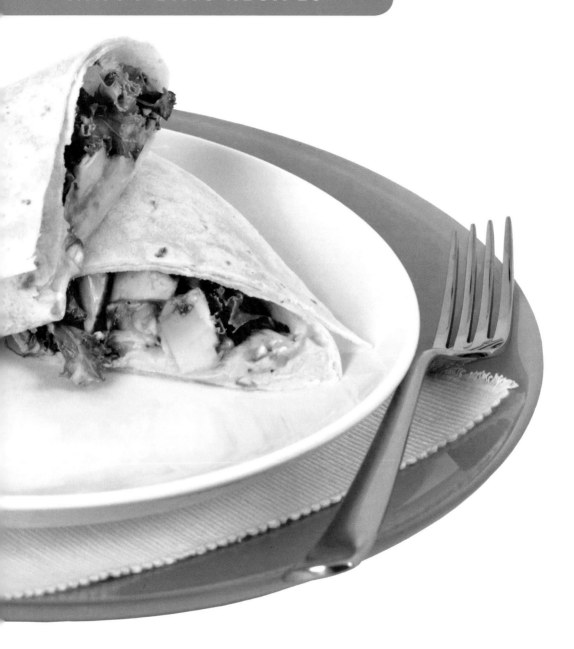

sweet kale wrap
184 SUGAR CALORIES, not 486 calories

¼ cup kale, chopped finely

5 cubes mango, ½" each

1 tsp. jalapeño, minced

1 Tbsp. mushrooms, chopped

1 Tbsp. balsamic vinegar

½ Tbsp. olive oil

1 whole-wheat tortilla

2–3 Tbsp. hummus

¼ avocado, sliced

Salt and pepper

In a small bowl, toss together the kale, mango, jalapeño, mushrooms, balsamic vinegar, and olive oil; season with salt and pepper. Spread the tortilla with hummus, top with salad mixture, and add avocados. Roll and eat.

VEG yes

VGN yes

D yes

G use La Tortilla Factory Smart & Delicious Gluten-Free Wrap

S yes

QUICK TIP

You can also use chopped spinach in place of the kale.

feta turkey burger

120 SUGAR CALORIES, not 400 calories

1 turkey patty
¼ cup spinach
2 Tbsp. feta cheese
1 whole-wheat hamburger bun
1 Tbsp. real mayonnaise
½ cup mixed greens
Olive oil
Red wine vinegar
Salt and pepper

Heat broiler to high. Season each side of burger with salt and pepper. Spray a broiler pan with nonstick spray (line with foil for an easier clean up), and place burger under broiler. Broil each side for 4–6 minutes, until no longer pink inside. Add feta, and return under broiler for just a minute, until cheese begins to melt. Spread mayo on bun, top with burger and spinach. Serve with mixed greens drizzled with olive oil and vinegar; season with salt and pepper.

QUICK TIP

Turn this burger into a patty melt. Add some sautéed onions and use Swiss cheese in place of the feta. Toast 2 slices of sourdough and use in place of the bun.

VEG   replace patty with BOCA Original Vegan Burger

VGN   replace patty with BOCA Original Vegan Burger

D   omit feta cheese

G   replace bun with Udi's Gluten-Free Classic Hamburger Bun

S   yes

citrus shrimp

90 SUGAR CALORIES, not 391 calories

5 medium shrimp

1–2 Tbsp. lime juice

¼ cup black beans (canned are fine, rinsed and drained)

½ cup cooked rice, brown is best

Olive oil

Salt and pepper

Shredded lettuce or spinach

Heat grill or broiler on high, brush shrimp with olive oil, and season with salt and pepper. You can skewer the shrimp if it makes them easier to handle on the grill. Place in the broiler or on the grill, and cook 2 minutes on each side until pink throughout. Toss shrimp with lime juice, rice, and beans, and adjust salt and pepper to taste. Serve on a bed of lettuce or spinach.

QUICK TIP

You can also use pinto or kidney beans in place of the black beans.

VEG you can substitute five 1" cubes of tofu fried in peanut oil until browned on all sides, drained on paper towels, and seasoned with salt and pepper

VGN see above

D yes

G yes

S substitute sliced chicken breast

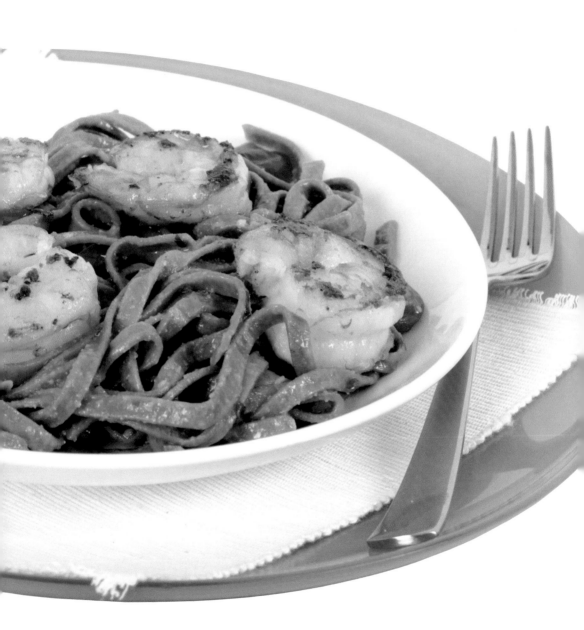

spinach pasta with shrimp

53 SUGAR CALORIES, not 200 calories

¾ cup spinach pasta, cooked

4 medium shrimp

3 cherry tomatoes, sliced

1 Tbsp. fresh parsley, chopped

Olive oil

½ garlic clove, minced

Dash red pepper flakes

Salt and pepper

Heat grill or broiler on high, brush shrimp with olive oil, and season with salt and pepper. You can skewer the shrimp if it makes them easier to handle on the grill. Place in the broiler or on the grill, and cook 2 minutes on each side until pink throughout. Toss with pasta, tomatoes, parsley, garlic, and red pepper flakes. Drizzle with olive oil, and season with salt and pepper.

VEG omit shrimp or use tofu as described in Citrus Shrimp recipe

VGN omit shrimp, or use tofu as described in Citrus Shrimp recipe

D yes

G use Lundberg Brown Rice Pasta

S substitute grilled chicken strips for shrimp

QUICK TIP

I love to add a little chopped spinach to this dish and top with a sprinkle of Parmesan.

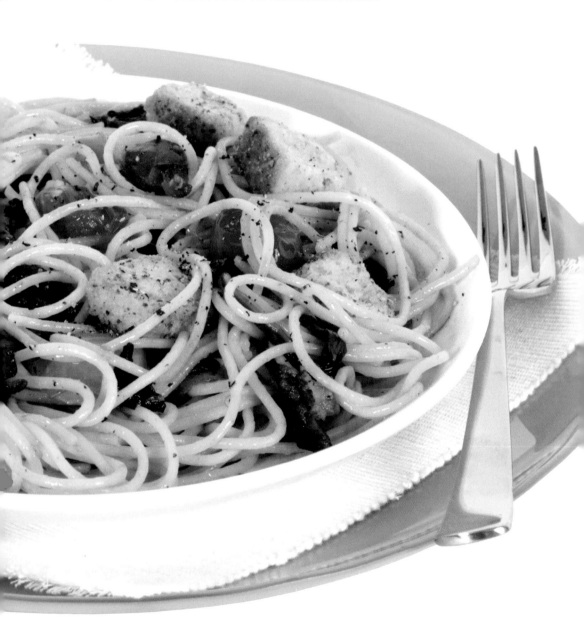

bacon spaghetti with garlic croutons

168 SUGAR CALORIES, not 375 calories

¾ cup whole-wheat spaghetti, cooked

1 strip bacon

3 cherry tomatoes, cut in half

¼ cup spinach, chopped

Olive oil

5 garlic croutons

Salt and pepper

Cook bacon according to package directions, and drain on paper towels. In a bowl, toss together the pasta, crumbled bacon, tomatoes, and spinach. Drizzle with olive oil, and season with salt and pepper. Top with croutons.

QUICK TIP

Serve on a bed of chopped spinach or arugula for extra greens, and omit pasta if you want to cut some sugar calories.

VEG replace bacon with Lightlife Smart Bacon

VGN replace bacon with Lightlife Smart Bacon

D yes

G use Lundberg Spaghetti Brown Rice Pasta; use Boar's Head Bacon; use Gillian's Foods Garlic Croutons

S yes

chicken spanish wrap

80 SUGAR CALORIES, not 488 calories

1 chicken breast

Olive oil

1 whole-wheat tortilla

2 Tbsp. black beans (canned is fine, rinsed and drained)

2 Tbsp. cooked rice

1 Tbsp. chopped onions

1 Tbsp. fresh cilantro, chopped

1 Tbsp. tomato, chopped

1 Tbsp. cheddar cheese

¼ avocado, sliced

Salt and pepper

Heat grill or broiler on high. Brush chicken with olive oil, and season with salt and pepper. Place chicken in broiler or on grill, and cook until no longer pink inside and juices run clear, about 10 minutes each side. When done, slice chicken thinly. In a bowl, toss together the beans, rice, onions, cilantro, and tomato. Put chicken on wrap, followed by bean mixture, and topped with cheese and avocado. Roll and eat.

QUICK TIP

This dish makes a great on-the-go lunch. Cook the filling ahead of time, and store in a container in the fridge. When ready to eat, put in a tortilla and roll.

VEG omit chicken and increase black beans to ½ cup

VGN omit chicken and cheese, increase black beans to ½ cup, and add 1 Tbsp. chopped walnuts

D omit cheese, and add 1 Tbsp. chopped walnuts

G use La Tortilla Factory Smart & Delicious Gluten-Free Wrap

S yes

italian chicken pita

150 SUGAR CALORIES, not 454 calories

½ chicken breast

1 whole-wheat pita

2 slices provolone cheese

1 Tbsp. marinara sauce (no sugar added)

1–2 Tbsp. fresh basil, chopped

¼ cup spinach, chopped

Salt and pepper

Heat grill or broiler on high. Brush chicken with olive oil, and season with salt and pepper. Place chicken in broiler or on grill, and cook until no longer pink inside and juices run clear, about 10 minutes each side. When done, slice chicken thinly. Fill pita with chicken, marinara, basil, spinach, and cheese; season with salt and pepper.

QUICK TIP

You can also replace the pita with ¾ cup whole-wheat pasta, cooked according to directions and tossed with the rest of the ingredients.

VEG replace chicken with Beyond Meat Chicken-Free Strips

VGN omit cheese and add 1 Tbsp. of chopped walnuts; replace chicken with Beyond Meat Chicken-Free Strips

D omit cheese and substitute 1 Tbsp. of chopped walnuts

G use La Tortilla Factory Smart & Delicious Gluten-Free Wrap

S yes

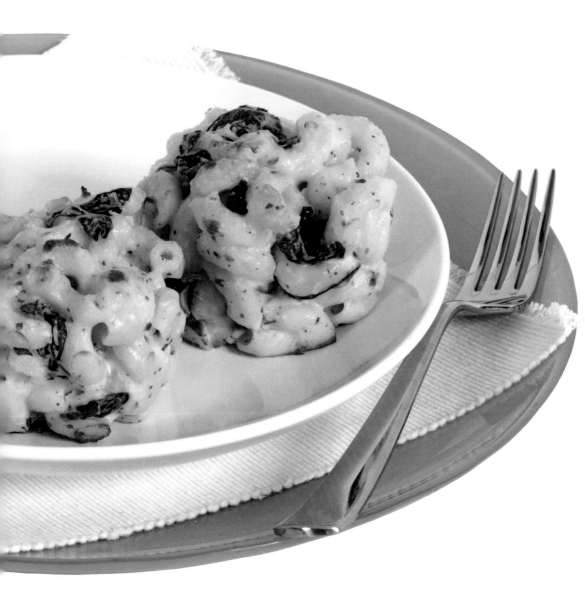

spinach macaroni bites

148 SUGAR CALORIES, not 413 calories

1 tsp. butter

1 tsp. almond flour

¼ cup half-and-half

¼ garlic clove, minced

¼ cup mozzarella cheese, shredded

1 egg, lightly beaten

1 cup whole-wheat macaroni noodles, cooked

1 cup fresh spinach, chopped

Nonstick cooking spray

Salt and pepper

Preheat oven to 400°F, and spray two muffin tins with cooking spray. In a saucepan, melt the butter over medium heat, then add the almond flour, half-and-half, garlic, egg, and cheese; season with salt and pepper. Stir until melted, then turn off heat and stir in cooked macaroni and spinach. Pour equal amounts of the noodle mixture into the two muffin tins, and bake in the middle of oven for 10–15 minutes, or until slightly golden.

QUICK TIP

This is a good recipe to multiply and freeze. Then, on a busy night, you can pop these little bites out and reheat in the microwave for 2 minutes.

VEG yes

VGN replace butter with Earth Balance Natural Buttery Spread; replace half-and-half with unsweetened almond milk; replace cheese with Daiya Mozzarella Style Shreds; replace egg with Ener-G Egg Replacer

D replace butter with Earth Balance Natural Buttery Spread; replace half-and-half with unsweetened almond milk; replace cheese with Daiya Mozzarella Style Shreds

G substitute Lundberg Elbow Brown Rice Pasta for the macaroni

S yes

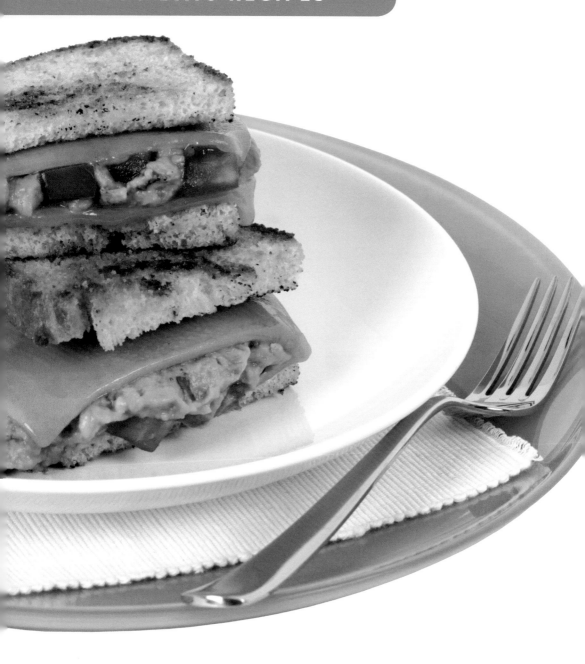

guacamole grilled cheese

120 SUGAR CALORIES, not 522 calories

2 slices cheddar cheese

¼ tomato, chopped

2 Tbsp. avocado, mashed

1 Tbsp. salsa

1 tsp. lemon juice

2 slices crusty whole-grain bread, toasted

Butter

Salt and pepper

In a small bowl, mash the avocado, stir in the lemon and salsa, and season with salt and pepper. Heat a cast-iron or nonstick skillet and melt about 2 tsp. of butter. While the skillet is heating, build your sandwich in this order: slice of toast, slice of cheese, avocado mixture, tomatoes, salt and pepper, the final slice of cheese, and the last slice of toast. Put the whole thing in the skillet, and heat each side until the cheese is melted. Don't be afraid to press down slightly with a spatula while grilling. **Note:** Feel free to use a panini press to fix this sandwich as well.

QUICK TIP

Use a whole-wheat tortilla and make this into a quesadilla. Skip the toasting, and put the tortilla in a heated skillet with the topping on one half. Fold, and brown each side until cheese melts.

VEG yes

VGN replace cheese with Tofutti American Soy-Cheese Slices; replace butter with Earth Balance Natural Buttery Spread

D replace cheese with Tofutti American Soy-Cheese Slices; replace butter with Earth Balance Natural Buttery Spread

G use Udi's Gluten-Free Whole Grain bread

S yes

chicken stir-fry

99 SUGAR CALORIES, not 377 calories

Olive oil

½ garlic clove, minced

½ Tbsp. fresh ginger, minced

2 Tbsp. onion, chopped

¼ cup broccoli, cut into bite-size pieces

¼ carrot, sliced into long strands

1 boneless chicken breast, cut into bite-size pieces

Salt and pepper

½ cup rice, cooked

Put a deep skillet over high heat; add half the olive oil and swirl it around, then add the garlic and ginger. Cook for about 20 seconds, then add the onion and cook for 2 minutes more. Add the broccoli and carrots and cook until crisp-soft, about 5 minutes. Turn the heat down to low, and remove the vegetables to a bowl.

Add another drizzle of olive oil to the pan, turn the heat to high, then add the chicken. Toss and stir the chicken until it has lost its pink color, about 5 minutes. Add the vegetables back into the chicken, then add the soy sauce, and salt and pepper to taste. Stir until most of the liquid is absorbed, just a minute or two more. Serve over cooked rice.

QUICK TIP

This dish is also delicious if made with shrimp or thinly sliced steak.

VEG   replace chicken with Beyond Meat Chicken-Free Strips

VGN   replace chicken with Beyond Meat Chicken-Free Strips

D   yes

G   yes

S   yes

pig in a wrap

86 SUGAR CALORIES, not 245 calories

2 slices of bacon

½ diced tomato

½ cup romaine lettuce, shredded finely

2 tsp. mayonnaise

1 whole-wheat tortilla

Salt and pepper

Heat a cast-iron or nonstick skillet and cook bacon according to package directions. Drain on paper towels. Heat your tortilla in the microwave for 30 seconds, then spread with mayo and top with crumbled bacon, tomato, lettuce, and salt and pepper.

QUICK TIP

Use chopped spinach in place of romaine for a heartier green.

VEG   replace bacon with Lightlife Smart Bacon

VGN   replace mayonnaise with mashed avocado; replace bacon with Lightlife Smart Bacon

D   replace mayonnaise with mashed avocado

G   use La Tortilla Factory Smart & Delicious Gluten-Free Wrap

S   yes

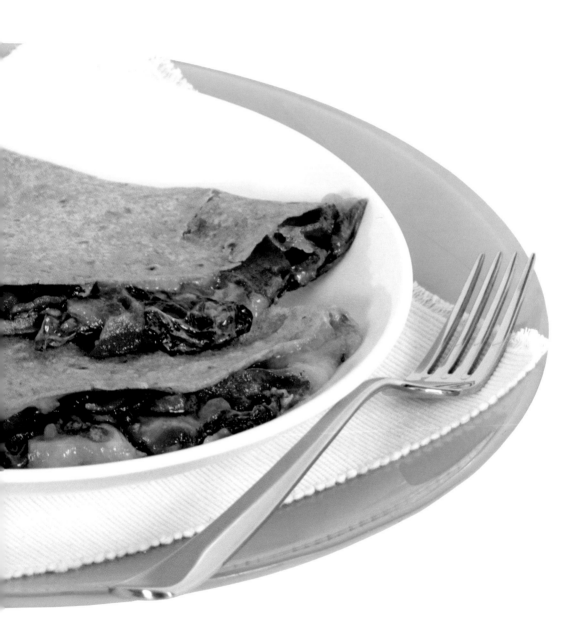

spinach bacon quesadilla

82 SUGAR CALORIES, not 290 calories

1 whole-wheat tortilla

1 Tbsp. cream cheese

½ cup spinach, chopped

2 slices bacon

1 Tbsp. cheddar cheese, grated

1 tsp. butter

Salt and pepper

Heat a cast-iron or nonstick skillet on medium-high and cook bacon according to package directions, then remove to paper towels to drain. On one half of the tortilla, spread the cream cheese and top with crumbled bacon, spinach, cheddar cheese, and salt and pepper. Fold tortilla in half and add to the skillet where you cooked the bacon, and cook on each side until brown and cheese is melted.

QUICK TIP

For less mess, you can also cook bacon in the microwave. Line a microwave-safe dish with a couple paper towels and place your bacon on top. Cover with one more sheet of paper towel. Microwave on high for 2–3 minutes, until done.

VEG replace bacon with Lightlife Smart Bacon

VGN replace cream cheese with Follow Your Heart Vegan Gourmet Cream Cheese; replace bacon with Lightlife Smart Bacon; replace cheese with Daiya Cheddar Style Shreds; replace butter with Earth Balance Natural Buttery Spread

D replace cream cheese with Follow Your Heart Vegan Gourmet Cream Cheese; replace cheese with Daiya Cheddar Style Shreds; replace butter with Earth Balance Natural Buttery Spread

G use Mission Corn Tortillas

S yes

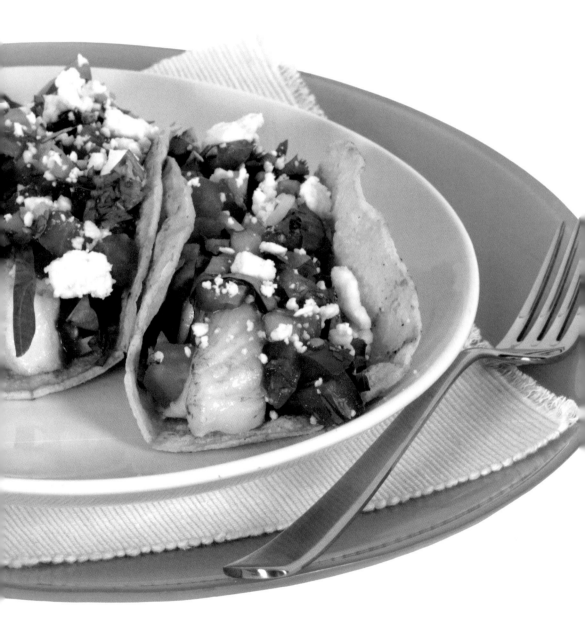

mediterranean tacos

54 SUGAR CALORIES, not 314 calories

1 mahi mahi fillet

2 Tbsp. feta cheese, crumbled

1 Tbsp. onion, chopped

2 tsp. fresh basil, chopped

2 Tbsp. pico de gallo

Salt and pepper

2 small corn tortillas

Heat a nonstick skillet on medium-high and add a drizzle of olive oil. Meanwhile, season the fish with salt and pepper on both sides. When the oil is hot, but not smoking, add the fillet and cook for 3 minutes, then turn and cook for another 3 minutes. Heat the corn tortillas in a skillet, then top with fish, cheese, and vegetables. Season with salt and pepper.

QUICK TIP

You can also heat a whole-wheat tortilla and roll up the filling for a handy wrap.

VEG   replace fish with Quorn Naked Chik'n Cutlet

VGN   replace fish with Quorn Naked Chik'n Cutlet, and omit cheese

D   replace cheese with Daiya Pepperjack Style Shreds

G   use Mission Corn Tortillas

S   replace fish with grilled chicken breast

pesto pita pizza

70 SUGAR CALORIES, not 315 calories

½ whole-wheat pita (cut so you have the round)

I tsp. pesto

I Tbsp. mozzarella, shredded

I chicken breast, grilled and sliced

I Tbsp. black olives, chopped

I Tbsp. fresh basil, chopped

I tsp. Parmesan

Salt and pepper

Preheat oven to 425°F. Spread the pita with pesto and top with the chicken, olives, basil, mozzarella, and Parmesan; season with salt and pepper. Bake on baking sheet or pizza stone for 10–12 minutes, until cheese is melted.

QUICK TIP

You can also use a whole-wheat tortilla in place of the pita—cook as directed above. Or make it a wrap: put the filling in a heated tortilla, and roll.

VEG replace chicken with Beyond Meat Chicken-Free Strips

VGN replace chicken with Beyond Meat Chicken-Free Strips; omit cheese and use Tofutti, Daiya, or another brand of dairy-free cheese; omit pesto and use marinara sauce

D omit cheese and use Tofutti, Daiya, or another brand of dairy-free cheese; omit pesto and use marinara sauce

G use Udi's Gluten-Free Whole Grain tortilla

S yes

tuna melt

60 SUGAR CALORIES, not 456 calories

½ can tuna, drained
1–2 Tbsp. mayonnaise
½ celery stalk, chopped
Salt and pepper
1 slice whole-grain toast
2 slices cheddar cheese

Mix together the tuna, mayonnaise, and celery; season with salt and pepper. Put filling on top of toast and top with cheddar cheese. Place under broiler until cheese is melted.

QUICK TIP

Put this filling in a whole-wheat tortilla and make it a wrap. Or skip the bread altogether and serve on top of a bed of chopped spinach with 5–10 garlic croutons and lemon wedges.

VEG substitute mashed tofu in place of tuna

VGN substitute mashed tofu in place of tuna

D yes

G use Udi's Gluten-Free Whole Grain bread

S substitute mashed tofu or canned chicken in place of tuna

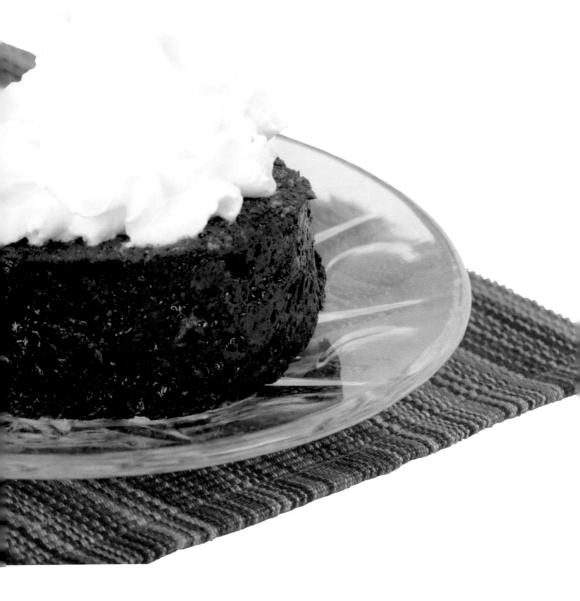

2-minute cake

0 SUGAR CALORIES, not 207 calories

(MAKES 4 SERVINGS)

¼ cup Truvia Baking Blend (Vons carries this)
½ cup almond flour (see tip below)
3 Tbsp. unsweetened cocoa powder
⅛ tsp. baking powder
½ tsp. baking soda
¼ tsp. salt
2 Tbsp. coconut oil
1 egg
2 Tbsp. half-and-half
1 cup whipping cream
1 packet of Truvia

In a bowl, mix together the dry ingredients. In another bowl, mix together wet ingredients, and then combine the dry mixture into the wet. Put ¼ of the batter into a coffee mug and microwave on high for 1 minute. Whisk together whipping cream and Truvia packet until thickened. Top cake with cream. Refrigerate remaining batter for later use.

QUICK TIP

If you can't find almond powder, pulse almonds in a coffee grinder or food processor until they become a flour-like consistency. (Be careful not to overprocess them into paste.)

VEG yes

VGN omit whipping cream; replace egg with Ener-G Egg Replacer; replace half-and-half with So Delicious Unsweetened Coconut Milk or something similar

D use unsweetened soy creamer in place of half-and-half; omit whipping cream

G yes

S yes

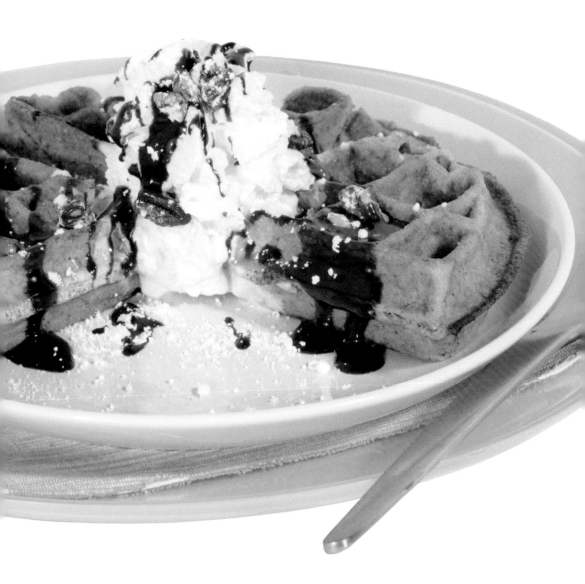

sweet skinny waffle

0 SUGAR CALORIES, not 546 calories

You can go to www.skinnywaffle.com to purchase these premade, no–Sugar Calorie waffles. Pop them in the toaster, then top with whipped cream, stevia, and Barlean's The Essential Woman Chocolate Mint Swirl (www.barleans.com).

Additional toppings to try:

- cinnamon (0 Sugar Calories)
- unsweetened cocoa powder (0 Sugar Calories)
- nuts, such as pecans, almonds, and macadamia nuts (0 Sugar Calories)
- Barlean's Omega Swirl, Key Lime (0 Sugar Calories)
- Barlean's Omega Swirl, Lemon Zest (0 Sugar Calories)
- Barlean's Omega Swirl, Mango Peach (0 Sugar Calories)
- Barlean's Omega Swirl, Piña Colada (0 Sugar Calories)
- Barlean's Omega Swirl, Strawberry Banana (0 Sugar Calories)
- Barlean's Omega Swirl, Blackberry (0 Sugar Calories)
- ¼ sliced banana (27 Sugar Calories)
- ¼ cup blueberries (22 Sugar Calories)
- 3 cherries (16 Sugar Calories)
- 1 Tbsp. graham cracker crumbs (17 Sugar Calories)

Want to make them yourself? Here's how:

¼ cup coconut flour

1 Tbsp. unsweetened almond milk

2 tsp. cinnamon

1 Tbsp. Truvia Baking Blend

¼ tsp. baking powder

¼ tsp. sea salt

1 Tbsp. coconut oil

4 eggs

Nonstick cooking spray

Preheat waffle iron. Mix all ingredients well in a bowl. Spray waffle iron with cooking spray, then pour half the batter into the warm iron. Cook until golden brown. Remove from iron, and repeat with remaining batter.

6

week 5 and beyond

Congratulations! You've made it through the first four weeks of this plan. My guess, however, is that you might be peeking ahead to this chapter before your four weeks are actually up—and that's great! I'm all about looking ahead, because people who are forward thinkers are more likely to thrive, according to scientific research on motivation and success. So, whether you're ready to take these steps now or you just want to strategize for the future, you'll find useful suggestions in this chapter.

The four-week plan you just completed was highly structured to make your weight loss as effortless as possible. It was also designed scientifically for your life stage to help boost your mood and motivation to fuel healthy eating and steady weight loss. Now, at Week 5 and beyond, it's time to make some choices, which I will outline in the next pages.

Whatever you decide, consider sharing your success at JorgeCruise.com or Facebook.com/HappyHormonesSlimBelly and help cheer others on.

Strategy 1: Let Me Be Your Coach

If you are busy or would like more variety, you can get more menus and recipes at my website HappyHormonesSlimBelly.com. This makes for effortless dieting because I do all the work for you with my online program. I'll provide you with a new menu each week, so you'll have plenty of variety and never get bored. Plus, you'll always have access to delicious easy-to-make foods that follow the Happy Hormones, Slim Belly™ plan. Studies have shown that when people are coached they are able to triple their weight-loss results. That is the main reason I have developed this online resource where I can be your coach, giving you new recipes and meal planners and taking the stress out of weight control. If you are serious about making changes that last, come see what my online program has to offer you.

Strategy 2: Let This Book Coach You

You can also simply return to the first four weeks in Chapter 4 and follow the menus again. You already know the plan, you've bought the ingredients before, and the recipes are easy—your brain doesn't have to do overtime. There is great power in simplicity, which can be a huge bonus in our busy lives. If you enjoy a structured routine and don't mind repeats, you may find that following the guidelines in this book and knowing exactly what to eat each week is a perfect fit for your lifestyle. Use the recipes as a mix-and-match resource: the Sugar Calories are already counted for you, and any Happy Day recipe can be swapped for another (and the same goes for Slim Day recipes).

Strategy 3: You Be the Coach

You can read on and learn how to take your new knowledge to the next level and start making your own menus from the food lists located in Chapter 7. To create your own meals and menus, review the following blank planners. All you have to remember is that Slim Days are 100 Sugar Calorie days—so you choose mostly foods that fall under the Freebie Foods lists in the next chapter. Alternately, on Happy Days, you make the choice to eat up to 500 Sugar Calories, a combination of foods found on the Freebie Foods and Sugar Calorie lists in the next chapter.

For the fastest weight loss, choose the healthiest Sugar Calories (high-fiber whole grains), try to stay under 100 Sugar Calories a day, and save the foods with the highest levels of sugars and refined flours for special treat days. In addition, make sure you include plenty of Freebie Vegetables from the lists on page 232. The high fiber in the foods will help you feel full and satisfied, so you lose weight faster. Refer back to Chapter 4 for on-the-go suggestions for each plan, as well as tips for checking in with your emotions to see whether you should choose to eat Slim (100 Sugar Calories) or Happy (up to 500 Sugar Calories) on a particular day.

For the Most Rapid Weight Loss

If after four weeks on the Happy Hormones, Slim Belly™ program, you find that your moods have leveled out and your carb and sugar cravings have been eliminated, then I highly recommend that you try my program The 100™. It works by having you eat 100 Sugar Calories or less a day. You will recognize this strategy as the Extra-Slim Plan in this book because it is based on The 100™ plan, the details of which you can find online at 100SugarCalories.com and in my book *The 100™*.

The 100™ is scientifically proven to provide the most rapid weight-loss results because it dramatically lowers insulin to liberate fat from your fat cells. With my book and online club, you will have access to hundreds of menus and recipe ideas that help you stick to 100 Sugar Calories or less per day.

That said, many women, especially those aged 40 to 60, continue to experience mood fluctuations as well as carb and sugar cravings. If this is your experience, then I encourage you to stick with my Carb Cycling Plan. You will continue to experience steady, moderate weight loss and long-term success.

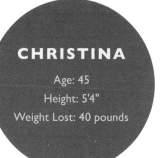

CHRISTINA
Age: 45
Height: 5'4"
Weight Lost: 40 pounds

I had been on one diet or another for the last decade, but my weight wasn't budging. Worse than that, in the last year I'd noticed that my belly was getting bigger no matter what I tried to do or how much I starved myself. On Jorge's plan I never felt hungry, but I still lost 10 pounds the first week!

BEST STRATEGY:

Splitting my meals and always having snacks on hand. I find that I do best if I portion my food into 6 small servings a day. I also keep baggies of pumpkin seeds in my purse and car, so I don't give in to an unhealthy snack while I'm out and about.

BIGGEST CHALLENGE:

Sugar cravings. They still hit me sometimes, usually at night when I watch TV. Thankfully, I can feed my sweet tooth and still stay on track with this plan. I'm sure to keep a little dark chocolate on hand, and a square or two seems to do the trick for me.

GREATEST PAYOFF:

The positive ripple effect: I eat right, which makes me feel better, which makes me want to get off the couch and go out. Plus my doctor noticed my complexion was glowing, and he commented that I seemed happy. Best of all: My skinny jeans are now loose!

YOUR PLANNER

The Carb Cycling Plan is based on 2 Slim Days (on consecutive days of your choosing) and 5 Happy Days. The Extra-Happy Plan is 7 Happy Days, and the Extra-Slim Plan is 7 Slim Days. Keeping this in mind, use the planner that matches your day of eating.

In the first column, track your meals: write down what you're eating and the amounts. In the second column, mark whether or not the food is a Freebie Food. Finally, in the third column, write down the amount of Sugar Calories in each food. (To calculate your Sugar Calories, look at the nutrition label and multiply the total carbohydrate grams by 4.)

Slim Day Planner

On Slim Days, you'll choose foods mostly from the Freebie Foods lists in Chapter 7, but can eat up to 100 Sugar Calories per day. Use the following planner on these days.

MEAL: BREAKFAST	FREEBIE FOOD	SUGAR CALORIES
MEAL: SNACK	FREEBIE FOOD	SUGAR CALORIES
MEAL: LUNCH	FREEBIE FOOD	SUGAR CALORIES
MEAL: SNACK	FREEBIE FOOD	SUGAR CALORIES
MEAL: DINNER	FREEBIE FOOD	SUGAR CALORIES
MEAL: TREAT	FREEBIE FOOD	SUGAR CALORIES
TOTAL SUGAR CALORIES FOR DAY (keep under 100)		

Happy Day Planner

Remember that you can choose up to 500 Sugar Calories on a Happy Day. The fewer Sugar Calories you have, the more rapidly the weight will come off—but keep in mind that if you are feeling low, it is better to have more Sugar Calories (up to 500) than to set yourself up for a sugar binge.

MEAL: BREAKFAST	FREEBIE FOOD	SUGAR CALORIES
MEAL: SNACK	FREEBIE FOOD	SUGAR CALORIES
MEAL: LUNCH	FREEBIE FOOD	SUGAR CALORIES
MEAL: SNACK	FREEBIE FOOD	SUGAR CALORIES
MEAL: DINNER	FREEBIE FOOD	SUGAR CALORIES
MEAL: TREAT	FREEBIE FOOD	SUGAR CALORIES
TOTAL SUGAR CALORIES FOR DAY (keep under 500)		

SMART CARB
BREAKFAST AND SNACKS

For days when you're feeling down or blue, give yourself an extra serotonin boost by eating a carb-only breakfast and an afternoon carb snack (see the bulleted list below for suggestions). Based on the latest research, this works best if you start your day with one of the suggested carb breakfasts listed below, then have protein (such as a small handful of almonds) for your snack 3 hours later, then have a protein/vegetable lunch 3 hours after that, then have a carb snack 3 hours after, and then eat a protein/vegetable dinner 3 hours after your afternoon nosh. Finally, if you're going to have a treat at the end of the day, make it a low-carb option. Timing-wise, it would look something like this:

7 a.m.: 2 pieces of sourdough or whole-grain toast with half of a mashed banana

10 a.m: Small handful of almonds

1 p.m.: Salad with chicken, and dressing of your choice

4 p.m.: 3 cups popcorn, salted (no butter)

7 p.m.: Grilled fish or steak with steamed or sautéed veggies of your choice (and butter)

9 p.m.: 2-Minute Chocolate Cake (see on page 215)

CARB BREAKFAST IDEAS:

- 2 slices of toast with mashed banana and sprinkle of cinnamon
- Cream of Wheat (made with water) with ¼ cup blueberries
- Oatmeal (made with water) with ½ chopped apple
- 2 slices of toast with sugar-free fruit spread

CARB SNACK IDEAS:

- 9 Triscuits
- 3 cups popcorn, salted, no butter
- 15 tortilla chips

Nonfood Happy Hormone Boosters

There are several ways to boost the hormones and neurotransmitters that control your mood that aren't related to food. Remember that if you're feeling bluer than usual, having carb or sugar cravings, or find yourself falling into emotional eating, it is probably an indicator that your serotonin levels are lower than they should be. To boost your serotonin, try any of the following activities. Try to do one or more of these every day, especially when you're feeling extra low. Here's a list of them:

— **Massage.** While it's great to get a professional massage on a regular basis, a freebie works just as well. Trade a 20-minute shoulder or back rub with a significant other or a close friend to elevate serotonin levels. To find a certified massage therapist in your area, visit www.amtamassage.org/findamassage/index.html.

— **Meditation.** Who would've thought that sitting and doing nothing could have such tremendous benefits for your health? It's true, though, mindfulness mediation yields improvements in health that range from lowering blood pressure to eliminating depression. This act of simply sitting and focusing on your breath will also boost your serotonin. I recommend doing this for 5 to 15 minutes every day. There are myriad meditations available to listen to online, on your phone, or on your iPod. One of my favorites is an audiobook available on iTunes called *Mindfulness Meditation: Nine Guided Practices to Awaken Presence and Open Your Heart* by Tara Brach. Whenever I have a few minutes to spare, I can pop on my headphones and meditate just about anywhere.

— **Gardening.** This activity raises your endorphins and your serotonin due to the exercise you get from weeding, mowing, and raking, as well as simply exposure to the sun. You can find gardening classes at local plant nurseries, community colleges, and adult learning centers. Go on, get your hands dirty!

— **Knitting.** Research has shown that repetitive activities, such as knitting, crocheting, or sewing, increase levels of serotonin. It's also a good way to keep your hands busy and out of the candy bowl. If you don't know how, you can call a local fabric or yarn shop; many of them have classes.

— **Chewing gum.** Yep, scientific research shows that chewing gum increases serotonin. Just be moderate, and go for varieties without sugar or dangerous artificial sweeteners (xylitol-sweetened ones are fine). And remember, chew with your mouth closed, please.

— **Playing music.** Music is magic. Research shows that it overrides stressors in the brain and body, releases endorphins, and increases the manufacturing of serotonin. You can get this benefit from picking up a guitar or just putting on some tunes. Either way, take a music break at least once a day.

— **Playing board games.** Social activities and games increase serotonin. After dinner, instead of heading toward the tube, pull out a board game and sit down with your family. Scrabble, Apples to Apples, and Scattergories are great choices, but if you have younger kids, Chutes and Ladders and Candyland work just as well.

— **Laughing.** This is the most fun you'll have boosting serotonin. Tune in to a good comedy, search for "laughing babies" on YouTube, or head out to a local standup comedy or improv club to get your fix.

— **Yoga and tai chi.** These ancient exercises are often referred to as moving meditations (and I already told you what meditation can do for you). Pairing gentle concentrated stretches and movements with a focused mind and deep breathing will optimize your serotonin levels. Check out your local gym, community college, or even church for classes.

— **Sunshine.** Not only will 20 minutes in the sun boost your vitamin D, it will release mood-improving endorphins and boost serotonin. Pair it with a walk, and you'll get double the payback.

— **Sleep.** Aim to get at least 7 to 9 hours of sleep every night. Being sleep deprived causes serotonin to plummet and sets you up for binges. Make your bedroom a sleep refuge by banning electrical devices and covering any lights. Even the glare of an alarm clock can keep sleep hormones from working effectively. Insomnia experts also recommend that you aim to keep the same sleep hours night after night, just like you tell your kids to do. This repetition helps your body know when it's time for rest and makes it easier to sleep.

MAGNESIUM MAGIC

Magnesium is the fourth most abundant mineral in the human body. It helps maintain normal muscle and nerve functions, regulates blood sugar levels, promotes a healthy blood pressure, and is involved in energy metabolism and protein synthesis. Magnesium is also intimately related to serotonin; when one is low, so is the other. So, by default, making sure you get enough magnesium in your diet is a good way to ensure that your serotonin levels stay high enough to keep you happy. The best way to get enough magnesium is to eat plenty of dark leafy greens, nuts, and whole grains. In the following chart, you'll find a list of foods that have the highest amounts of this nutrient. The menus in Happy Hormones, Slim Belly™ are designed to include at least 320 milligrams of magnesium per day (the recommended daily amount for women over 30). When you move beyond the first four weeks and begin designing your own menus, keep this in mind. It's one of the reasons I often include almonds as a daily snack.

FOOD	MILLIGRAMS	DAILY VALUE
Almonds, dry roasted, 1 oz.	80	20%
Avocado, ½ cup	22	6%
Banana, 1 medium	32	8%
Black-eyed peas, cooked, ½ cup	46	12%
Brown rice, long-grain, cooked, ½ cup	42	11%
Cashews, dry roasted, 1oz.	74	19%
Kale, raw, 2 cups	63	16%
Kidney beans, canned, ½ cup	35	9%
Lentils, cooked, ½ cup	36	9%
Nuts, mixed, dry roasted, 1oz.	64	16%
Oatmeal, instant, 1 cup	61	15%
Peanut butter, 2 Tbsp.	49	12%
Peanuts, dry roasted, 1 oz.	50	13%
Pinto beans, cooked, ½ cup	43	11%
Potato, with skin, baked, 1 medium	48	12%
Soybeans, cooked, ½ cup	74	19%
Spinach, cooked, ½ cup	78	20%
Spinach, raw, 2 cups	47	12%
Whole-wheat bread, 1 slice	23	6%

7

the food lists

The Happy Hormones, Slim Belly™ lists of foods are found on the following pages. The concept is simple when planning and organizing your meals for the week: On Slim Days, or if you are following the Extra-Slim Plan, you want to choose foods that are mostly from the Freebie Foods lists. This avoids most Sugar Calories, keeping your insulin as low as possible and releasing belly fat and weight from your body the fastest. You do get to eat up to 100 Sugar Calories per day, but you do not have to use your entire allotment. (As previously mentioned, this strategy follows my plan for most rapid weight loss, The 100™.) Alternatively, on Happy Days, or if you use the Extra-Happy strategy, you'll choose foods from all lists, tracking to be sure that you don't go over 500 Sugar Calories per day. This is easy with the following Happy Hormones, Slim Belly™ lists, because I've done the math for you.

These are not exhaustive lists. To use an item that is not on the food lists that follow, you'll just need to read the nutrient label on the side of the package. You can calculate any food's Sugar Calories from the grams of carbohydrates listed on the nutrient label. To determine the number of Sugar Calories in a particular food, all you have to do is multiply the number of total carbohydrate grams by 4. It's simple math. (However, you can also visit HappyHormonesSlimBelly.com for a more extensive list of Sugar Calorie calculations.)

THE FREEBIE FOODS

These foods don't need to be counted as they do not cause significant spikes in insulin. (However, always check the nutrition labels of packaged foods, as brands do vary and some may contain added sugar.)

PROTEINS

POULTRY

Chicken breast

Cornish hen

Duck

Goose

Pheasant (no skin)

Rotisserie chicken
(my favorite is Costco's brand, Kirkland Signature)

Turkey bacon

Turkey breast

Turkey burger

Turkey, lean ground

EGGS

Chicken (brown or white)

Duck

Egg whites

Goose

SEAFOOD

Catfish

Clams

Cod

Crab

Flounder

Halibut

Lobster

Mahi mahi

Orange roughy

Oysters

Salmon

Sardines

Scallops

Shrimp

Sole

Swordfish

Tilapia

Trout

Tuna

RED MEAT & PORK

Bacon

Beef (trimmed of fat), including:

  chuck

  cubed

  flank

  ground

  jerky

  porterhouse

  rib

  round, sirloin

  rump roast

  T-bone steak

  tenderloin

Bierwurst or beer-wurst

Bologna

Buffalo

Canadian bacon

Capicola

Chorizo

Corned beef

Devon (sausage)

Ham

Hot dog

Lamb chop, leg, or roast

Liverwurst

Pastrami

Pepperoni

Pork center loin chop

Pork roll

Pork tenderloin

Prosciutto

Roast beef

Roast pork

Salami

Sandwich/deli meats

  - chicken

  - ham

  - roast beef

  - turkey

Sausage

Smoked meat

Summer sausage

Veal loin chop or roast

OTHER PROTEIN SOURCES

Almonds

Almond butter, unsweetened

Almond flour/meal

Brazil nuts

Cashews

Chick'n Strips, Meal Starter, Morningstar Farms

Hot dogs, Smart Dogs, Lightlife

Jay Robb Whey Protein

Macadamia nuts

Pecans

Pine nuts

Pumpkin seeds

Seitan

Sunflower seeds

Tempeh

Tofu

Veggie burgers, such
as Garden Veggie
Patties, Morningstar
Farms

Walnuts

VEGETABLES & FRUITS

Alfalfa spouts

Artichokes

Arugula

Asparagus

Avocado

Bell pepper, red, yellow,
orange, or green

Bok choy, regular or
baby

Broccoli

Brussels sprouts

Cabbage

Cauliflower

Celery

Collards

Cucumber

Eggplant

Endive

Fennel

Green beans

Green onion

Kale

Lemon

Lettuce, iceberg

Lettuce, red leaf

Lettuce, romaine

Lime

Mushrooms

Mustard greens

Okra

Onion

Pepper, jalapeño

Pepper, serrano

Pickles, dill

Radicchio

Radishes

Scallions

Seaweed

Shallots

Snap peas

Spinach

Summer squash

Swiss chard

Tomato

Turnip greens

Watercress

Zucchini

HERBS & SPICES (FRESH OR DRIED)

Basil	Ginger	Peppermint
Chives	Oregano	Salt
Cilantro	Parsley	Thyme
Garlic	Pepper	

FATS

Animal fats	Extra virgin olive oil (my favorite is Costco's brand, Kirkland Signature)	Sesame oil
Avocado oil		Walnut oil
Butter	Flaxseed oil	Any of Barlean's Omega Swirl flavors
Coconut oil	Ghee	

DAIRY PRODUCTS

CHEESE

American	Colby Jack	Fontina
Asiago	Cottage cheese	Gorgonzola
Blue	Cream cheese	Gouda
Brick	Dry Jack	Gruyère
Brie	Edam	Havarti
Cheddar	Farmer cheese	Limburger
Colby	Feta	Mascarpone

Monterey Jack	Pepper Jack	Scamorza
Mozzarella	Provolone	String cheese
Muenster	Queso blanco	Swiss
Parmesan	Ricotta	Teleme
Pepato	Romano	

OTHER

| Half-and-half | Plain Greek yogurt (FAGE Total brand, recommended) | Sour cream |
| | | Whipped cream |

MISCELLANEOUS

Almond milk, unsweetened	Coffee, black	Skinny Waffle™
Baking powder	Espresso	Soy cheese
Baking soda	Flax meal/flour	Soy milk, unsweetened
Balsamic vinegar	Hot sauce	Soy sauce
Barlean's Forti-Flax	Italian dressing	Sparkling water
Blue cheese dressing	Mayonnaise	Stevia
Chia flour	Mustard	Stevita Tropical Singles (flavored stevia drink packs)
Coconut flakes, unsweetened	Ranch dressing	Tea, unsweetened, hot or iced
Coconut flour	Raw Chocolate Drink	
Coconut milk, unsweetened	Salsa	Truvia
	Sesame seeds	Vinegar
	Skinny Maple Syrup™	Water

SUGAR CALORIES

I have created a list of many common foods that are important to count toward your daily allowance of Sugar Calories. If a food is not listed below, but is not on the Freebie Foods list, make sure to look up the total carbohydrate amount and multiply by 4 to get the Sugar Calorie total.

DAIRY PRODUCTS

Milk, 1% or fat free (1 cup) = 49 SUGAR CALORIES

Milk, nonfat dry (⅓ cup) = 12 SUGAR CALORIES

Milk, whole (1 cup) = 51 SUGAR CALORIES

Rice milk, plain, Rice Dream (1 cup) = 92 SUGAR CALORIES

Soy milk, plain, Silk (1 cup) = 32 SUGAR CALORIES

Yogurt, fat-free plain (6 oz.) = 52 SUGAR CALORIES

LEGUMES

Baked beans, original, Bush's Best (¼ cup) = 116 SUGAR CALORIES

Black beans, cooked (½ cup) = 92 SUGAR CALORIES

Chickpeas (garbanzo beans) (½ cup) = 65 SUGAR CALORIES

Edamame, shelled (soybeans) (½ cup) = 40 SUGAR CALORIES

Hummus (2 Tbsp.) = 16 SUGAR CALORIES

Kidney beans (¼ cup) = 40 SUGAR CALORIES

Lentils (¼ cup) = 40 SUGAR CALORIES

Pinto beans (¼ cup) = 44 SUGAR CALORIES

CARBOHYDRATES

BREADS AND TORTILLAS

Bagels, honey whole wheat (1) = 224 SUGAR CALORIES

Bread, sprouted whole grain (1 slice) = 60 SUGAR CALORIES

Bread, whole wheat (1 slice) = 88 SUGAR CALORIES

Hamburger bun (1) = 72 SUGAR CALORIES

Hamburger bun, sprouted whole grain (1) = 136 SUGAR CALORIES

Pancakes, plain frozen, ready-to-heat (4" diameter; 1) = 60 SUGAR CALORIES

Pita, whole wheat (1) = 62 SUGAR CALORIES

Roll, small dinner (1) = 52 SUGAR CALORIES

Tortilla, corn (6" diameter; 1) = 23 SUGAR CALORIES

Tortilla, flour (6" diameter; 1) = 64 SUGAR CALORIES

Waffles, frozen, ready-to-heat (4" diameter; 1) = 60 SUGAR CALORIES

Wrap, organic whole wheat (1) = 80 SUGAR CALORIES

PASTA

Penne, whole wheat, cooked (1 cup) = 208 SUGAR CALORIES

Spaghetti, whole wheat, cooked (1 cup) = 151 SUGAR CALORIES

Spirals, whole wheat, cooked (1 cup) = 149 SUGAR CALORIES

CEREALS AND GRAINS

Cereal, Cheerios (¾ cup) = 72 SUGAR CALORIES

Cereal, Ezekiel 4:9 sprouted whole grain (½ cup) = 160 SUGAR CALORIES

Cereal, Ezekiel 4:9 sprouted whole grain golden flax (½ cup) = 148 SUGAR CALORIES

Cereal, Post shredded wheat (1 cup) = 164 SUGAR CALORIES

Cereal, Total (¾ cup) = 92 SUGAR CALORIES

Cereal, Uncle Sam's (¾ cup) = 152 SUGAR CALORIES

Cereal, Wheaties (¾ cup) = 88 SUGAR CALORIES

Corn-muffin mix, "Jiffy" (¼ cup) = 108 SUGAR CALORIES

Couscous, cooked (½ cup) = 73 SUGAR CALORIES

Granola, low-fat (½ cup) = 160 SUGAR CALORIES

Oatmeal, dry steel cut (¼ cup) = 108 SUGAR CALORIES

Oatmeal, Quaker original instant (1 packet) = 76 SUGAR CALORIES

Oatmeal, Quaker instant apples and cinnamon (1 packet) = 88 SUGAR CALORIES

Quinoa, cooked (½ cup) = 79 SUGAR CALORIES

Rice, basmati, cooked (½ cup) = 88 SUGAR CALORIES

Rice, brown, cooked (½ cup) = 92 SUGAR CALORIES

Rice, jasmine, cooked (½ cup) = 106 SUGAR CALORIES

Rice, Spanish, cooked (½ cup) = 80 SUGAR CALORIES

Rice, white, cooked (½ cup) = 106 SUGAR CALORIES

VEGETABLES

Corn, yellow (½ cup) = 58 SUGAR CALORIES

French fries, fast food (1 large) = 260 SUGAR CALORIES

Potato (1 medium) = 146 SUGAR CALORIES

Rutabaga, cubes (1 cup) = 58 SUGAR CALORIES

Sweet potato (1 medium) = 92 SUGAR CALORIES

Turnip, cubes (1 cup) = 34 SUGAR CALORIES

Vegetable blend, stir fry frozen (¾ cup) = 20 SUGAR CALORIES

Winter squash, acorn (½ cup) = 75 SUGAR CALORIES

Winter squash, butternut (½ cup) = 43 SUGAR CALORIES

Yam (½ cup) = 75 SUGAR CALORIES

F R U I T S

Fruits have lots of vitamins and can be a healthy part of any diet. However, they are primarily carbohydrates and natural sugar, so we do need to pay attention to how much we consume because they spike insulin. Some experts say that the sugar and carbs in fruit don't count because they're offset by the fiber and water content, but others say that it can still affect weight loss. I suggest choosing fruit with the fewest Sugar Calories and keeping servings to no more than two a day.

Apple (I medium) = 99 SUGAR CALORIES

Apricot (I medium) = 16 SUGAR CALORIES

Banana (I medium) = 108 SUGAR CALORIES

Banana, dried (¼ cup) = 240 SUGAR CALORIES

Blackberries (½ cup) = 29 SUGAR CALORIES

Blueberries (½ cup) = 43 SUGAR CALORIES

Cantaloupe, cubed (½ cup) = 29 SUGAR CALORIES

Cherries (9) = 47 SUGAR CALORIES

Grapefruit, red and pink (½) = 21 SUGAR CALORIES

Honeydew (I wedge) = 46 SUGAR CALORIES

Kiwi (I medium) = 40 SUGAR CALORIES

Mango, sliced (½ cup) = 52 SUGAR CALORIES

Orange (I small) = 45 SUGAR CALORIES

Peach (I medium) = 59 SUGAR CALORIES

Pear (I small) = 92 SUGAR CALORIES

Pineapple, diced (½ cup) = 43 SUGAR CALORIES

Plum (1 medium) = 30 SUGAR CALORIES

Raspberries (1 cup) = 59 SUGAR CALORIES

Strawberries (1 cup) = 44 SUGAR CALORIES

Tangerines (1 medium) = 47 SUGAR CALORIES

Watermelon, diced (1 cup) = 46 SUGAR CALORIES

SNACKS & TREATS

Cheetos jumbo cheese puffs (1 oz.) = 60 SUGAR CALORIES

Doritos nacho cheese chips (1 oz.) = 68 SUGAR CALORIES

Granola bars, oats, fruits & nuts (1 bar) = 88 SUGAR CALORIES

Green and Black's organic 85% dark chocolate (12 pieces) = 60 SUGAR CALORIES

Ice cream, soft serve, vanilla (½ cup) = 70 SUGAR CALORIES

Joseph's Cookies, chocolate chip or oatmeal (4 cookies) = 52 SUGAR CALORIES

Kettle Chips, lightly salted (1 oz.) = 76 SUGAR CALORIES

Kettle corn (1 cup) = 100 SUGAR CALORIES

Nabisco Ritz Crackers, original (5) = 40 SUGAR CALORIES

Nabisco Wheat Thins multi-grain crackers (6) = 88 SUGAR CALORIES

Newman's Own chocolate crème cookies (2 cookies) = 80 SUGAR CALORIES

Pepperidge Farms goldfish crackers (55 pieces) = 80 SUGAR CALORIES

Pirate's Booty (1 oz.) = 72 SUGAR CALORIES

Popchips, original (22 chips) = 80 SUGAR CALORIES

Popcorn, air popped (3 cups) = 75 SUGAR CALORIES

Quaker rice cakes, lightly salted (2) = 56 SUGAR CALORIES

Trail mix (1 oz.) = 45 SUGAR CALORIES

Wasa Original Crispbread (2 pieces) = 80 SUGAR CALORIES

BEVERAGES

Apple juice (8 oz.) = 116 SUGAR CALORIES

Beer, Coors Light (1 bottle) = 20 SUGAR CALORIES

Beer, Michelob Ultra (1 bottle) = 10 SUGAR CALORIES

Beer, Miller Lite (1 bottle) = 13 SUGAR CALORIES

Beer, O'Doul's, nonalcoholic (1 bottle) = 53 SUGAR CALORIES

Energy drink, Diet Rockstar (8 oz.) = 8 SUGAR CALORIES
(but contains dangerous artificial sweeteners)

Energy drink, Red Bull, sugar free (8 oz.) = 11 SUGAR CALORIES
(but contains dangerous artificial sweeteners)

Ginger ale, Schweppes (4 oz.) = 46 SUGAR CALORIES

Grapefruit juice, light, Ocean Spray (8 oz.) = 120 SUGAR CALORIES

Orange juice (8 oz.) = 104 SUGAR CALORIES

Soda, Diet Coke (8 oz.) = 0 SUGAR CALORIES
(but contains dangerous artificial sweeteners)

Soda, Steaz, organic sparkling green tea (1 can) = 92 SUGAR CALORIES

Sports drink, Gatorade, lemonade (4 oz.) = 30 SUGAR CALORIES

Vegetable juice, V8 100% (8 oz.) = 40 SUGAR CALORIES

Wine, dessert (1 glass, 3 oz.) = 80 SUGAR CALORIES

Wine, red (1 glass, 3 oz.) = 14 SUGAR CALORIES (my favorite is Kirkland Signature cabernet sauvignon)

Wine, white (1 glass, 3 oz.) = 15 SUGAR CALORIES (my favorite is Kirkland Signature chardonnay)

CONDIMENTS & DRESSINGS

Apple sauce, unsweetened (½ cup) = 56 SUGAR CALORIES

Barbecue sauce (2 Tbsp.) = 102 SUGAR CALORIES

Cocktail sauce (2 Tbsp.) = 30 SUGAR CALORIES

Honey (1 Tbsp.) = 69 SUGAR CALORIES

Ketchup (1 Tbsp.) = 15 SUGAR CALORIES

Miracle Whip, light (2 Tbsp.) = 24 SUGAR CALORIES

Peanut butter (2 Tbsp.) = 25 SUGAR CALORIES

Ranch dressing (2 Tbsp.) = 8 SUGAR CALORIES

Teriyaki sauce (2 Tbsp.) = 28 SUGAR CALORIES

Xylitol crystals (1 Tbsp.) = 24 SUGAR CALORIES

FROZEN FOODS

Amy's Frozen Meals

Black Bean and Vegetable Enchilada = 88 SUGAR CALORIES

Mexican Tofu Scramble = 160 SUGAR CALORIES

Shepherd's Pie = 108 SUGAR CALORIES

Spinach Feta Pocket Sandwich = 136 SUGAR CALORIES

Lean Cuisine Frozen Meals

Alfredo Pasta with Chicken & Broccoli = 180 SUGAR CALORIES

Baked Chicken = 120 SUGAR CALORIES

Beef Pot Roast = 104 SUGAR CALORIES

Chicken and Vegetables = 116 SUGAR CALORIES

Chicken Marsala = 116 SUGAR CALORIES

Garlic Beef and Broccoli = 172 SUGAR CALORIES

Glazed Chicken = 116 SUGAR CALORIES

Grilled Chicken Caesar Bowl = 132 SUGAR CALORIES

Lemongrass Chicken = 140 SUGAR CALORIES

Meatloaf with Gravy & Whipped Potatoes = 100 SUGAR CALORIES

Roasted Chicken with Lemon Pepper Fettuccini = 112 SUGAR CALORIES

Roasted Garlic Chicken = 44 SUGAR CALORIES

Roasted Turkey & Vegetables = 72 SUGAR CALORIES

Rosemary Chicken = 108 SUGAR CALORIES

Salisbury Steak with Mac & Cheese = 92 SUGAR CALORIES

Salmon with Basil = 100 SUGAR CALORIES

Shrimp Alfredo = 112 SUGAR CALORIES

Shrimp and Angel Hair Pasta = 136 SUGAR CALORIES

Steak Tips Portobello = 56 SUGAR CALORIES

Stuffed Cabbage = 112 SUGAR CALORIES

Swedish Meatballs = 140 SUGAR CALORIES

8

the blissful workout

T he biggest misconception about exercise, working out, lifting weights, and fitness is that it can be the be-all and end-all solution to weight loss. I've talked a lot about the misguided advice that is mainstreamed to the masses, and exercise for weight loss is another component of the conventional wisdom touted by the media, health officials, and government agencies—but it just isn't true.

You can't lose weight and keep it off by simply hitting the treadmill, going to spin class, or hoisting weights. And while this might sound like bad news, it isn't. Moving your body is still an essential component in any healthy lifestyle, and it will certainly help you lose weight, feel better, and look better faster. The trick is to make sure to implement exercise in the way your body was meant to work on a biological level, just like your eating habits. When you address and use exercise in this way, it becomes your best friend on the quest to slim down and be happy, and to stay that way for a lifetime.

Exercise alone can't cause weight loss—the harder you work out, the more your body works to replace the lost calories. Remember, your body is always striving to maintain balance, and this system is the same when it comes to exercise, especially long, intense sessions of exercise. Say you head into spin class and have a sweat-drenching hour of brutal hill climbs and sprints. You may burn 500 or more calories, but this places your body in an immediate state of imbalance. The message your cells get postexercise is "Replenish—quickly." Chemical messengers are sent out that stimulate your appetite, spurring you to replace the calories you just burned off, as well as encouraging you to conserve energy by moving less.

All this might lead you to think, *Well, then, I should just lounge around on the sofa all day*—but not so quick, my friend. Equilibrium-supporting exercise is a whole different matter. If you use physical activity in a way that supports your genetic blueprint, it will become your best friend. Exercise is actually one of the most important supporting agents for women over 40 who are trying to lose weight. Done right, exercise can double the hormones and neurotransmitters that keep you feeling your most motivated and inspired to stick with your weight-loss plan. Moving your body for just a few minutes a day can double your serotonin levels and increase energy-revving norepinephrine. According to new research from the *British Journal of Sports Medicine,* exercise also increases the chemical messengers that ramp up your self-control and make you impervious to cravings. On a practical level, exercise will distract you from your worries, lower your levels of stress, increase your fat-burning abilities for the following 24 hours, and improve the way you look. The best news is, you'll see the greatest results when exercise is enjoyable, fun, and short. Here's how to put it to your best use.

QUALITY, NOT QUANTITY

I recommend that you find some enjoyable way of moving your body each and every day. If you haven't been active at all, then start with just 5 minutes of walking a day. Work up to 10 minutes, then aim for 20. If you feel like doing more, great—but 20 minutes of gentle movement every day is all you need to increase serotonin, improve your mood, and keep cravings at bay. In the rest of this chapter, I'll go through other exercises you might include as you see fit to ramp up your weight loss.

Moving to Ramp Up Motivation

Research shows that exercise works as well as antidepressants when it comes to improving mood, lowering stress, and increasing energy. Different types of exercise offer different benefits. Knowing how the following can help you feel and look your best, and how to use them for their maximum benefit, is key. Here's the breakdown:

1. Moving meditations. To lower stress, boost your body's disease-fighting system, and increase your serotonin, consider checking out a relaxing yoga or tai chi class. These fitness strategies work by combining concentration, breathing, and gentle movements. You'll also improve flexibility and strength. Many gyms and community centers offer such classes. Do a quick Google search for your area and check out a class, or go on YouTube and look up easy workout routines.

2. Strength training. If you are looking to decrease flabbiness and increase fitness and muscle tone, it is far better to spend less time on the treadmill and more time lifting weights or doing sit-ups and push-ups. The great part about doing strength training is that you will build muscle and increase fat burning, which will make your body look and feel more toned and trim. But, in addition, doing a short strength-training routine (as in "The Happy Hormones, Slim Belly™ Workout" on the next page) can double your levels of serotonin and increase the hormones that ramp up your energy.

3. Walking. Putting one foot in front of the other is probably the easiest way to ramp up your feel-good hormones and neurotransmitters, especially if you stroll in the sun. In just 20 minutes of walking, your body increases serotonin, endorphins that lower stress, and the energy-raising norepinephrine. At the same time, the sun *also* ramps up your production of serotonin and endorphins, and increases your body's production of vitamin D, which lowers disease and improves mood. And there's research to show that walking in nature, or even in a neighborhood that has trees and flowers, lowers stress and improves mood.

4. Dancing. I never want exercise to be something you stress about, because that defeats the purpose, which is increasing your self-control, lowering stress, and improving your mood. The key is to keep it low-key and fun. With this in mind, consider simply plugging in your iPod and playing some of your favorite music (especially on busy days). You can boogie even as you're making dinner—and trust me, you'll feel happier in just a few minutes. Music overrides many of the blocks we carry around in our heads that keep us feeling stressed and overwhelmed. Pairing tunes with a little fun movement is a great way to break through common stressors.

5. Social exercise. Another trick to giving your serotonin a boost while lowering stress is to invite others to join you in an activity, such as taking a Zumba class, biking with the family, taking a hike with some friends, and even walking the dog. This has been shown to spike serotonin and reduce stressors. These sessions get you out of your own head, and besides, you'll be a great role model to those around you, which will also increase your commitment to your goals.

THE HAPPY HORMONES, SLIM BELLY™ WORKOUT

You can double your levels of serotonin, ramp up your energy-revving hormones, and release feel-good endorphins almost immediately with the following five moves. The best news? No gym and no equipment needed.

What you'll need: A comfortable carpeted space (or use a yoga mat or towel), and a good attitude.

What to do: Aim to do these five simple moves on four nonconsecutive days of the week. Many of my clients try to do them Monday, Wednesday, Friday, and Sunday. You can knock them all out in one 20-minute workout. You can do these moves on their own, or after you take a short stroll.

1. Waist whittler. Start from your hands and knees and then move into a push-up position, so that your body forms a straight line from your head to your heels. Look at the ground, but don't let your head sag. Keeping your abdominal muscles and back muscles tight, slowly bend your left knee and bring it to your left elbow, then return to start. Repeat this for 30 seconds. Then switch sides to repeat the movements on the right: bend your right knee and bring it to your right elbow, then return.

To make this move easier: Start from your hands and knees in a tabletop position.

To make this move harder: Bring your left knee to your right elbow, so it crosses underneath your body. Do this for 30 seconds. Then repeat on the other side, bringing your right knee to your left elbow.

2. Butt buster. Lie on your back on the floor. Keeping your back flat and your arms down along the sides of your torso, bend your knees and slide your feet in so that they are a couple of inches in front of your knees, flat on the floor. Squeeze your butt muscles as you press into your feet to raise your hips and your back off the floor. You should form a straight line from your shoulders to your knees. Hold for a second, and then slowly lower. Your feet and arms stay flat on the floor throughout the move. Repeat for 1 minute.

To make this move easier: Don't press your butt as high.

To make this move harder: Do the move with the left leg straight, so that it is in line with the right hip and knee—do the move for 30 seconds, then switch to the right foot extended, and do for another 30 seconds.

3. Shoulder shaper. Sit on the floor and place your feet, knees bent, flat on the floor in front of you. Place your hands several inches behind your butt with fingertips pointing toward your backside. Arms should be shoulder width apart. Press into your hands and feet to lift your butt and hips off the floor to form an upside-down tabletop position. Keeping your abdominals and back contracted and firm, bend your elbows to less than 90 degrees; hold for a second, then press back up. Repeat for 1 minute.

To make this move easier: Keep your butt on the ground and use the upper body as weight as you bend your elbows.

To make this move harder: Extend one leg and do the move for 30 seconds on one side, then switch legs and do 30 seconds on the other side.

4. Chest chiseler. Lie on your belly on the floor with your knees bent and your feet up in the air, ankles crossed. Place your hands by your shoulders and press up into a modified push-up position so that you form a straight line from your head to your knees. Walk your hands closer together so that your two pointer fingers touch and your thumbs touch, forming a diamond shape with your hands. Keeping your abdominals and your back firm, bend your elbows and lower your chest until you are a couple inches off the floor, then push back up. Repeat for 1 minute.

To make this move easier: Use a table to lean against and perform the move in an angled push-up position from the table.

To make this move harder: Perform this move from a traditional push-up position so that you are in a straight line from your head to your toes with your legs straight and lifted.

5. Thigh trimmer. Stand with your feet hip width apart and raise your arms straight in front of you, shoulder width apart, palms facing down. Lift your left foot and extend it a couple inches in front of you, keeping your leg straight. From this position, slowly squat down by bending your right knee and maintaining your balance. Keep your arms and left leg raised throughout the move. Hold for a second, then press back up. Repeat for 30 seconds, and then switch sides for a total of 1 minute.

To make this move easier: Place a chair to one side to use as support throughout the move.

To make this move harder: Do this move for a full minute on each side.

9

frequently asked questions (FAQs)

1. HOW DOES THE WOMEN'S CARB CYCLING™ PLAN CAUSE WEIGHT TO BE LOST SO SUCCESSFULLY?

The basic understanding is that cutting Sugar Calories for two days resets your insulin response and ultimately boosts your serotonin levels. When your body is reset, your insulin sensitivity increases, which means it takes less carbs (which you will eat on Happy Days) to satisfy your serotonin needs. The result is faster weight loss, because insulin levels are moderated, while serotonin levels are optimized so appetite stays sated, carb cravings are eliminated, and motivation is elevated.

2. HOW QUICKLY WILL I SEE CHANGES?

Clients of mine notice results almost immediately. Within the first two days, weight loss and a sense of renewal will come over you. After the first week the majority of my clients experience large amounts of weight loss, especially those who have more than 40 pounds to lose. Clients who had 15 to 20 pounds to lose experienced a 2- to 5-pound weight loss on average, but some lost up to 9. It all depends on your commitment and the amount you have to lose. I promise you this: stick to the plan as I have outlined, and you *will* see dramatic results!

3. DOES MY AGE MAKE WEIGHT LOSS DIFFICULT?

Absolutely. That is why this program was developed. In fact gender and age are the two biggest factors to consider when developing a program for weight loss. At this life stage, hormones are fluctuating, life in general can be more complicated, and stress is a daily part of life. The good news is that Happy Hormones, Slim Belly™ addresses all this in the best possible way to make sure your hormones are in check, your diet isn't something you stress about, and your serotonin is soaring, leaving you with a feeling of peace and bliss.

4. CAN I FOLLOW MORE THAN 2 SLIM DAYS?

You sure can, *if* you are able to stave off cravings and your mood stays elevated. When dipping into the third day of cutting Sugar Calories, it is important to check in with how you feel to make sure that you are not feeling irritable, sad, or lethargic, which often leads to cravings. Cravings can be the sabotage of weight loss, but you can keep them at bay by following a Happy Days menu until you feel more balanced. Those who have successfully curbed their cravings may want to check out my program The 100™, which helps you stick to this way of eating for a lifetime. See www.JorgeCruise.com/the100 for more information.

5. CAN I FOLLOW MORE THAN 5 HAPPY DAYS?

The truth is, anybody can follow the Happy Days of Happy Hormones, Slim Belly™ and still see results. However, detoxing from Sugar Calories for two days will give you even better results. My recommendation is that those who cannot curb their cravings and successfully stay away from Sugar Calories for two days, as well as women over 60 or who are in menopause, would benefit the most from consistently following the Belly Fat Cure™. See www.JorgeCruise.com/bellyfatcure for more information.

6. CAN MEN FOLLOW HAPPY HORMONES, SLIM BELLY™ AND LOSE WEIGHT AS WELL?

Yes. This diet will work for men as well as women. For couples, I'd suggest sticking together on the same diet plan for ease of use. However, since men don't deal with the same hormonal fluctuations as women, I'd recommend that they follow The 100™ for maximum results.

7. WHAT CAN I EAT WHEN I AM AWAY FROM THE KITCHEN?

I'd say that 99.9 percent of my clients are busy, and eating at home is not always an option. So when going to a restaurant or someplace that meals are made, I come prepared—not with food, but with a determination to stick to my plan. What I do is describe the meal that I want to have, or "order off the menu." I typically order something I know they will have—for example, a chicken salad with ranch or blue cheese dressing. I might also choose a lean protein option that is used on the menu, and ask for it grilled or steamed, with a double order of low-sugar vegetables in place of the usual starchy, carbohydrate-laden side dishes. Most establishments will be happy to help you stick to your healthful eating plan.

8. CAN I EAT AS MUCH I WANT OF FOODS THAT HAVE ZERO CARBS AND ZERO SUGARS, OR IS THERE A LIMIT?

Within reason, if a food contains no Sugar Calories—any Freebie Food, such as cheddar cheese—your goal should be to eat to satisfaction, not feeling stuffed. Be aware of your body—eat slowly, and if you feel full, stop eating.

9. DO I HAVE TO EAT ALL THE FOOD ON THE MENU EVERY DAY?

No. The rule of thumb is to always check in with how you are feeling. You want to eat when you are hungry and stop when you feel satisfied, not stuffed. That said, aim to get the vegetables that are listed on the meal planners because they provide high levels of antioxidants, vitamins, and minerals (especially magnesium) to boost your immune system and serotonin levels. Cut carbs first! If you feel full on a Happy Day menu, see if you might be satisfied with one less serving of toast or pasta. This will help your weight to come off faster as well.

10. WHAT DO I DO IF I STOP LOSING WEIGHT ON THE HAPPY HORMONES, SLIM BELLY™ PLAN?

Weight-loss plateaus happen for a variety of reasons. Sometimes it's merely a function of your body adjusting after you've had a few weeks of dramatic or moderate weight loss. In this case, the action you need to take is a lesson in patience—stick with the program as you've been doing, and continue to take your waist measurement. Often when you stop losing weight you are still losing inches, which is a sign that body fat is dropping off even if the scale doesn't register it.

At other times a stall in weight loss can be about your attention to detail. Maybe you've slipped a bit and are eating more sugars or too many carbs. For example, I recommend a maximum of 60 Sugar Calories per serving of bread, which many brands exceed. Remember to check the nutrition labels on all packaged and prepared foods. In this case, I suggest taking a close look at the foods you are eating. Write everything down for three days and make sure you are following at least two Slim Days a week.

If you've been following the Extra-Happy Menu, you may be getting more carbs than your body can handle when it comes to losing weight. In this case I suggest that you return to the recommended Carb Cycling menu or, if you feel like you can handle it, give the Extra-Slim Menu a try for a week (or even for three or four days) before going back to the Carb Cycling menu.

Finally, remember that if you're near your goal weight, those last few pounds will naturally be slow to come off your body, so be patient and stick with it—you'll get there!

11. DOES THIS PROGRAM ALLOW ME TO HAVE FRUIT?

The answer is yes; Happy Hormones, Slim Belly™ *lets* you enjoy fruit! First keep in mind that if your goal is truly to get rid of body fat, then you have to limit fruits because they have sugars in them—even though these are natural sugars, they can still spike your insulin levels if you eat too many of them per day, depending on your individual tolerance to carbs and sugars. Fructose, the sugar found in fruit, goes directly to the liver to be processed and gets converted to dangerous trigylcerides and free radicals. High fructose consumption also causes insulin resistance, which can lead to diabetes. Remember that fruit grew in warm climates and historically was available only certain times of the year. Today we have access to nearly any type of fruit every day of the year, which is not how our bodies are designed to consume fruit.

On your Happy Days you can enjoy up to 500 Sugar Calories, and I recommend that those Sugar Calories come from the best sources first; try using this as your guide, in descending order from most to least ideal:

1. Beans and legumes
2. Starchy vegetables
3. Whole grains
4. Fruits
5. Refined carbs (white bread, rolls, buns)
6. Condiments
7. Treats and desserts

My suggestion is that when you do enjoy fruit, try to eat local, seasonal fruit in its complete, natural form (with the skin on) whenever possible, and remember to minimize it in extremely high-sugar forms such as smoothies and juices. Also, berries tend to be the lowest in sugars and highest in fiber and antioxidants.

12. DO I HAVE TO EXERCISE TO LOSE WEIGHT?

No. Exercising is optional, and studies have shown that it can actually be counterproductive to weight loss. Research done at the University of Michigan revealed that typical forms of exercise don't burn enough calories to make a difference for weight-loss purposes. In fact, since exercise actually makes some people hungrier, it can make eating the right amount of food each day difficult. However, while exercise as a direct method of weight loss is not something I see as useful, I do believe that regular activity is an important adjunct to weight loss, especially for women over 40. This is because the right kind of exercise (walking in the sunshine, for example) can raise levels of feel-good hormones such as serotonin and dopamine, which improves impulse control, reduces appetite, and keeps you feeling happy and energized to stay on track. In addition, strength training builds muscle, which not only looks better on your body but also helps your body burn more fat; it also increases serotonin and gives you energy and vitality. I've included the best sort of exercise to use with the Happy Hormones, Slim Belly™ plan in Chapter 8.

13. WILL THIS PLAN WORK FOR MY WHOLE FAMILY, INCLUDING KIDS?

Definitely! Happy Hormones, Slim Belly™ is a healthy lifestyle for everyone in your family. Avoiding hidden sugars is important for overall health in children, teens, adults, and seniors, regardless of gender or body weight. Low-sugar, nutrient-rich foods are as beneficial for your kids as they are for you. It may be difficult to change your kids' minds about sugar if they have fallen into a habit of constantly eating sugary snacks, but you can start by leading by example. If you stop buying junk food, this reduces both your and *their* access to unhealthy options. It's a win-win situation. Then, get your kids involved by teaching them about the benefits of certain foods and letting them help you prepare snacks and meals. Your kids will be more interested in the foods they are eating if they help create the meals with you. Try to make cooking something fun you and your kids can enjoy together.

14. HOW CAN I SHARE WITH YOU ABOUT THE WEIGHT I'VE LOST?

I'm always eager to hear about the success my clients have on this program. I encourage you to share your story, along with before and after photos, on JorgeCruise.com and on my Facebook page: www.Facebook.com/JorgeCruise.

15. HOW LONG CAN I FOLLOW THIS PLAN?

For the rest of your life! Follow the Happy Hormones, Slim Belly™ four-week plan, and you can lose up to 7 pounds the first week and 2 pounds a week thereafter. Your weight loss will vary depending on what you weigh when you start, how much you have to lose, and your individual metabolism (your fat-burning engine). When you reach a healthy weight, your body will naturally plateau. Most of my clients are so thrilled with the results they see and how much better they feel that they continue to use these tools as part of a healthy lifestyle.

16. WHAT KINDS OF ARTIFICIAL SWEETENERS SHOULD I AVOID?

Many people believe that the solution to cutting out sugars, but still feeding your sweet tooth, is to use the many alternative sweeteners that are available. Unfortunately, this doesn't work out so well for your health, or your weight-loss goals. The big three to avoid are:

— *Aspartame (Equal and NutraSweet, blue packages).* This sweetener was discovered in the 1960s by a chemist who was working on an ulcer drug. Aspartame is found in thousands of food and drink products—specifically, diet sodas. Risks listed in scientific research include imbalances in your brain, migraines, mood disturbances, and insomnia. Aspartame has been linked to increased seizures, according to research in the journal *Environmental Health Perspectives*. This sweetener is common in diet sodas, many sugarless gums, and some "light" yogurts.

— *Sucralose (Splenda, yellow packages).* Discovered in 1976 by a grad student who had been told to "test" some compounds, but misunderstood and did a "taste" test instead. When he reported the sweetness, sucralose was born. This sweetener is found in more than 4,500 food products, including candy, ice creams, and beverages. Sucralose is 600 times sweeter than sugar, but its health effects are anything but sweet. Good levels of naturally occurring gut bacteria (which aid digestion and promote healthy bowel movements) are reduced 50 percent by average consumers of sucralose, according to a Duke University study.

— *Saccharin (Sweet'N Low, pink packets).* This is the oldest sugar substitute around. It was also discovered by a chemist in 1879 and became popular in the 1900s. In the 1970s saccharin was linked to bladder cancer in animal studies, according to research published in *Science*. Instead of this resulting in banning the product, saccharin packages were required to include labeling that warned consumers of the risk. This ban was removed in 2001 when the study was reviewed and found to be faulty. Still, scientists from many institutions, including the University of Illinois and Boston University, call for continued carcinogen warnings on saccharin based on "evidence" to suggest that it is cancer causing.

These sugar substitutes have been coined "excitotoxins," by some experts, which means that they act in your brain by "overexciting" or overstimulating neurons, causing degeneration and even death in important nerve cells. When too many nerve cells die, your nervous system begins to malfunction, and it can't communicate with other parts of your body. This can ultimately lead to nervous-system disorders such as Parkinson's disease, multiple sclerosis, and Alzheimer's disease.

17. ARE THERE ANY SAFE SWEETENERS?

So what can you have that is sweet to eat? The Happy Hormones, Slim Belly™ plan was designed to allow for sweets and treats, and my two favorite healthy sweeteners are stevia and xylitol, which can be found in health-food stores and many supermarkets today. Stevia is an herb originally from South America; it is calorie-free, does not spike blood sugar or insulin, and can be used for baking. Plus, stevia is sweeter than sugar, so small amounts are sufficient. The FDA has approved rebaudioside A, which is a refined stevia extract, for use in food and drink products.

Xylitol is a sugar alcohol that is virtually calorie-free, and it doesn't spike blood sugar. Contrary to its name, xylitol doesn't contain alcohol; it's actually a type of carbohydrate. The reason this carbohydrate doesn't count is that your body can't digest it (most will be excreted in your urine). I do recommend that you keep xylitol to a minimum because some people find it causes gas and bloating when eaten in excess, so limit it to no more than 100 grams per day.

There are actually three sugar alcohols you'll see in food products—here's the breakdown:

— *Xylitol.* A sugar alcohol extracted from the fiber of various fruits and vegetables.

— *Malitol.* A sugar alcohol that is popularly used in many baked goods, chocolates, and cookies. I have heard from some of my clients that this sugar alcohol can make them feel bloated. It's a harmless reaction, but an uncomfortable one, so you may want to adjust your intake of these foods.

— *Erythritol.* This sugar alcohol is known for causing less gastrointestinal disturbances, and is a good one to look for.

18. WHAT IS THE DIFFERENCE BETWEEN HAPPY HORMONES, SLIM BELLY™ AND OTHER LOW-CARB DIETS SUCH AS ATKINS?

Like many low-carb diets, Happy Hormones, Slim Belly™ limits carbs and cuts hidden sugars to control and limit insulin production, but the similarities stop there. Happy Hormones, Slim Belly™ is designed to cycle on a weekly basis to keep a woman's insulin at maximum sensitivity so that she needs less carbs to activate the serotonin-boosting benefits that keep women succeeding long-term on weight-loss goals. Unlike Atkins (or South Beach) there are no phases to Happy Hormones, Slim Belly™, and rather than being truly low carb, Happy Hormones, Slim Belly™ is more of a Low Glycemic Load Diet—because there are still carbs included most days of the week, they're just the high-fiber, nutrient-rich carbs that benefit your body the most by raising your interior fat-burning engine, while keeping insulin levels optimal.

Here are other major distinctions that make Happy Hormones, Slim Belly™ a more healthful, more effective weight-loss program:

— *No ketosis.* The main goal of Atkins and other stringent very low-carb diets is to induce ketosis, which is a state the body enters when it is severely restricted of carbo-hydrates from all sources. Dieters following Atkins often buy strips that they urinate on to test for ketosis, but you won't ever be doing that on Happy Hormones, Slim Belly™.

— *No dangerous artificial sweeteners.* Atkins relies heavily on the use of artificial sweeteners like sucralose, while Happy Hormones, Slim Belly™ eliminates this and all other unnatural and potentially harmful chemicals from your diet.

19. CAN I STILL DRINK ALCOHOL ON THIS PROGRAM?

You may have noticed that, unlike my earlier plans, the menus in this book don't include alcohol. In the past, I included wine as a daily treat option, but for women age 40 to 60 who are trying to lose weight, alcohol can be an impediment to success.

Alcohol is a combination of sugars, carbs, and alcohol (ethanol). Ethanol is devoid of nutritional value (it's actually considered a toxin) and goes straight to your liver to be processed. The leftover Sugar Calories can spike your insulin levels and increase your fat. Women over 40 are more susceptible to these effects than men or younger women. In addition, alcohol can lower inhibitions and increase food cravings, making it easier to give in to that bowl of chips or the bread basket at the restaurant. To optimize your weight-loss results, it's best to just skip the cocktails. That said, if it's a special occasion, go ahead and enjoy a glass of your favorite beverage—I recommend red wine for the antioxidant levels—just be mindful of the Sugar Calorie content.

20. CAN I BE A VEGAN OR VEGETARIAN ON THIS PROGRAM?

Yes. Anyone can do this program, and that's why I included vegetarian- and vegan-friendly symbols and options for modifying every recipe in Chapter 5. While I believe animals are the most preferred source of protein for the human body, you can simply substitute the meats and/or cheeses I recommend in my books for your own favorite vegan or vegetarian options. Many of these options are included in the Food Lists in Chapter 7.

21. CAN I DO HAPPY HORMONES, SLIM BELLY™ IF I'M FOLLOWING A GLUTEN-FREE DIET?

Yes. Since the program is based on a simple, clean way of eating, it can easily be adapted to be gluten-free. I encourage you to eat plenty of lean proteins and healthy fats. Be sure to check out the suggestions I've given at the end of every recipe in Chapter 5. My favorite gluten-free product is the Light Brown Rice Loaf from Ener-G Foods. Check out ener-g.com for nutrition labels to track your carb servings, and more information on this bread and some of their other gluten-free products.

22. IF I'M THIN I DON'T NEED TO WORRY ABOUT EATING THIS WAY, RIGHT?

Not true. There are people who are genetically destined to store less food as fat (in other words, they look skinny), even if they eat a diet high in Sugar Calories, but this doesn't mean they are healthier. We've known for a long time that there is a genetic component to being fat or thin. This is often seen in teenagers, and you might have even once commented, "I used to be able to eat anything when I was younger, but then it caught up with me." Just because you can eat junky foods without gaining weight doesn't mean those foods aren't adversely affecting health. You can still have high levels of heart-clogging fats from the overconsumption of sugary foods and refined starches.

This is especially concerning in teens because many younger men and women think that they can just catch up and eat healthy later in life, and parents often go along with this thinking. But in reality, teens who eat this way are laying the foundation for insulin resistance and glucose intolerance, which will make them more likely to struggle with obesity, diabetes, heart disease, cancer, and so on in the later years of their life. It's just that their bodies are growing and so fuel is being partitioned differently than it will be when they get older. So, thin or fat, we all need to reduce our intake of Sugar Calories to protect our health.

selected bibliography

Abbott, Elizabeth. *Sugar: A Bittersweet History*. London and New York: Duckworth Overlook.

Anderson, I.M. et al. 1990. "Dieting reduces plasma tryptophan and alters brain 5-HT function in women." *Psychological Medicine*. 20(4): 785–91.

Anson, M.R. 2003. "Intermittent fasting dissociates beneficial effects of dietary restriction on glucose metabolism and neuronal resistance to injury from calorie intake." *Proceedings of the National Academy of Sciences of the United States of America*. 100(10): 6216–20.

Avena, N.M., Rava, P., & Hoebel, B.G. 2008 "Evidence for sugar addiction: Behavioral and neuro-chemical effects of intermittent, excessive sugar intake." *Neuroscience and Biobehavioral Reviews*. 32(1):20–39.

Beulens, J.W.J., et al. 2007. "High Dietary Glycemic Load and Glycemic Index Increase Risk of Cardiovascular Disease Among Middle-Aged Women." *Journal of the American College of Cardiology*. 50(1):14–21.

Brehm, B.J., et al. 2003. "A Randomized Trial Comparing a Very Low Carbohydrate Diet and a Cal-orie-Restricted Low Fat Diet on Body Weight and Cardiovascular Risk Factors in Healthy Women." *The Journal of Clinical Endocrinology & Metabolism*. 88(4):1617–23.

Cahill, G.F., et al. 1959. "Effects of insulin on adipose tissue." *Annals of the New York Academy of Sciences*. Sept 25; 82:4303–11.

Cloud, J. 9 August 2009. "Why exercise won't make you thin." *Time*. Retrieved from www.time.com/time/printout/0,8816,1914974,00.html.

Cohen LS, Soares CN, Vitonis AF, Otto MW, Harlow BL. "Risk for new onset of depression during the menopausal transition: the Harvard study of moods and cycles." *Arch Gen Psychiatry*. Apr 2006;63(4):385–90.

Cohn, V. "A passion to keep fit: 100 million Americans exercising." *Washington Post.* 31 August 1980.

Cordain L, et al. 2000. "Plant-animal subsistence ratios and macronutrient energy estimations in worldwide hunter-gatherer diets." *American Journal of Clinical Nutrition.* 71(3):682–692.

Ebbeling, C.B., et al. 2012. "Effects of dietary composition on energy expenditure during weight-loss maintenance." *Journal of the American Medical Association.* 307(24): 2627–34.

European Food Information Council. "Carbohydrates." Retrieved on 01 July 2013 from www.eufic .org/article/en/expid/basics-carbohydrates.

Fernstrom, J.D. and Wurtman RJ. 1972. "Brain Serotonin Content: Physiological Regulation by Plasma Neutral Amino Acids." *Science.* 27 October 1972: Vol. 178 no. 4059 pp. 414–16. DOI: 10.1126/Science.178.4059.414.

Fernstrom, J.D. and Wurtman RJ. 1971. "Brain serotonin content: increase following ingestion of carbohydrate diet." *Science.* 174 (4013): 1023–25.

Fogelholm, M. & Kukkonen-Harjula, K. 2000. "Does physical activity prevent weight gain—a systematic review." *Obesity Reviews.* 1(2): 95–111.

Freeman EW, Sammel MD, Liu L, Gracia CR, Nelson DB, Hollander L. "Hormones and Menopausal Status as Predictors of Depression in Women in Transition to Menopause." *Arch Gen Psychiatry.* Jan 2004;61, no. 1:62–70.

Garcia, A.D. Chan, W.Y. 1996. "The role of the placenta in fetal nutrition and growth." *Journal of the American College of Nutrition.* 15(3): 206–22.

Gardner, C.D. et. Al. 2007. "Comparison of the Atkins, Zone, Ornish, and LEARN diets for change in weight and related risk factors among overweight premenopausal women: the A TO Z Weight Loss Study: a randomized trial." *Journal of the American Medical Association.* 298(2):178.

Haist, R.E. & Best, C.H. 1966. "Carbohydrate Metabolism and Insulin." *The Physiological Basis of Medical Practice, 8th edition.* Baltimore: Williams & Wilkins.

Halbreich U. "Role of estrogen in postmenopausal depression." *Neurology.* May 1997;48(5 Suppl 7):S16–9.

Hargrove, J.L. 2006. "History of the calorie in nutrition." *The Journal of Nutrition.* 136: 2957–61.

Harvard Public School of Health. "Carbohydrates: Good Carbs Guide the Way." Retrieved on 01 July 2013 from www.hsph.harvard.edu/nutritionsource/carbohydrates-full-story.

Harvie, M.N., et al. 2011. "The effects of intermittent or continuous energy restriction on weight loss and metabolic disease risk markers: a randomized trial in young overweight women." *International Journal of Obesity.* 35(5): 714–27.

Indiana University, Office of Science Outreach. 24 August 2010. "Obesity, Type 2 Diabetes, and Fructose." Retrieved from www.indiana.edu/~oso/Fructose/Consequences.html.

Johnson, R.K., et al. 2009. "Dietary Sugars Intake and Cardiovascular Health : A Scientific Statement From the American Heart Association." *Circulation.* Retrieved from http://circ.ahajournals.org /content/120/11/1011.full.pdf.

Kennedy, E.T., et al. 2001. "Popular Diets: Correlation to health, nutrition, and obesity." *Journal of the American Dietetic Association.* April; 101(4): 411–20.

Kraschnewski, J.L., et al. 2010. "Long-term weight loss maintenance in the United States." *International Journal of Obesity.* 2010 Nov; 34(11):1644–54.

Larsson S.C., Bergkvist L., and Wolk A. 2006. "Consumption of sugar and sugar-sweetened foods and the risk of pancreatic cancer in a prospective study." *American Journal of Clinical Nutrition.* 84(5):1171–76.

Leibel R.L., Rosenbaum M., & Hirsch J. 1995. "Changes in energy expenditure resulting from altered body weight." *New England Journal of Medicine.* 332(10):621–28.

Lewis GF, et al. 2002. "Disordered fat storage and mobilization in the pathogenesis of insulin resistance and type 2 diabetes." *Endocrine Reviews.* 23(2) 201–09. Retrieved from http://edrv.endojournals.org/content/23/2/201.full.pdf+html.

Maartens LW, Knottnerus JA, Pop VJ. "Menopausal transition and increased depressive symptomatology: a community based prospective study." *Maturitas.* Jul 25 2002;42(3):195–200.

Maher, T.J. & Wurtman, R.J. 1987. "Possible neurologic effects of aspartame, a widely used food additive." *Environmental Health Perspectives.* 75:53–57. Retrieved from www.ncbi.nlm.nih.gov/pmc/articles/PMC1474447/pdf/envhper00434-0053.pdf.

Malik VS & Hu FB. 2012. "Sweeteners and Risk of Obesity and Type 2 Diabetes: The Role of Sugar-Sweetened Beverages." *Current Diabetes Reports.* 12(2): 195–203.

Martin, A., et al. 2000. "Is advice for breakfast consumption justified? Results from a short-term dietary and metabolic experiment in young healthy men." *British Journal of Nutrition.* 84(3):337–44.

Minkin, Mary Jane; et al. 1997. *What Every Woman Needs to Know about Menopause.* Yale University Press.

Moyer, M.W. 2010, "Carbs against cardio: More evidence that refined carbohydrates, not fats, threaten the heart." *Scientific American.* May 2010. Retrieved from www.scientificamerican.com/article.cfm?id=carbs-against-cardio.

Newburgh, L.H. 1930. "The Nature of Obesity." *Journal of Clinical Investigation.* 8(2): 197–213. doi:10.1172/JCI100260.

Nishizawa et al. 1997. "Differences between males and females in rates of serotonin synthesis in human brain." *PNAS.* 1997 94 (10) 5308–13. Retrieved from www.pnas.org/content/94/10/5308.full.pdf+html.

O'Connell, J. and Hawkes, K. 1981. "Alyawara Plant Use and Optimal Foraging Theory." *In Hunter-Gatherer Foraging Strategies.* Edited by Bruce Winterhalder and Eric Smith. Chicago: University of Chicago Press.

Ohlson, M.A., et al. 1955. "Weight control Through Nutritionally Adequate Diets." *Weight Control: A Collection of Papers Presented at the Weight Control Colloquium.* Eppright et al eds., pg. 170–87.

Oz, M. (24 February 2011). Gary Taubes on *The Dr. Oz* Radio Show Discussing Why We Get Fat, Part I, [*The Dr. Oz Show*]. Retrieved from http://youtu.be/IMUGUZ3EEEo.

Payne JL. "The role of estrogen in mood disorders in women." *Int Rev Psychiatry.* Aug 2003;15(3):280–90.

Pennington, A.W. 1953. "Treatment of Obesity with Calorie Unrestricted Diets." *American Journal of Clinical Nutrition.* 1(5):343–348.

Pirozzo, S., et al. 2002. "Advice on low-fat diets for obesity." *Cochrane Database System Review.* (2):CD003640. DOI: 10.1002/14651858.

Reaven GM. "Banting lecture 1988. Role of insulin resistance in human disease." *Diabetes.* 1988; 37:1595–607.

Rosenbloom, S. 23 March 2010. "Calorie data to be posted at most chains." *The New York Times.* Retrieved from www.nytimes.com/2010/03/24/business/24menu.html?_r=0.

Samaha, F.F., et al. 22 May 2003. "A Low-Carbohydrate as Compared with a Low-Fat Diet in Severe Obesity." *The New England Journal of Medicine.* 348: 2074–81.

Schernhammer, E.S., et al. 2005. "Sugar-Sweetened Soft Drink Consumption and Risk of Pancreatic Cancer in Two Prospective Cohorts." *Cancer Epidemiology, Biomarkers & Prevention.* 14(9): 2098–2105.

Schulze MB, et al. 2004. "Sugar-sweetened beverages, weight gain, and incidence of type 2 diabetes in young and middle-aged women." *Journal of the American Medical Association.* Aug 25;292(8):927–34.

Soares CN, Taylor V. "Effects and Management of the Menopausal Transition in Women with Depression and Bipolar Disorder." *J Clin Psychiatry.* 2007;68 (suppl 9):16–21.

Steiner M, Dunn E, Born L. "Hormones and mood: from menarche to menopause and beyond." *J Affect Disord.* Mar 2003;74(1):67–83.

Taubes, G. 17 February 2011. "Is Sugar Toxic?" *The New York Times.* Retrieved from www.nytimes .com/2011/04/17/magazine/mag-17Sugar-t.html?_r=0#.

Taubes, G. 2007. *Good Calories, Bad Calories: Fats, Carbs, and the Controversial Science of Diet and Health.* New York: Anchor Books.

Taubes, G. December 2011. *Why We Get Fat: And What to Do about It.* New York: Anchor Books.

Thomson, E.A. 20 February 2004. "Carbs are essential for effective dieting and good mood, Wurtman says." *MIT News.* Retrieved from http://web.mit.edu/newsoffice/2004/carbs.html.

Trapp, E.G., et al. 2008. "The effects of high-intensity intermittent exercise training on fat loss and fasting insulin levels of young women." *International Journal of Obesity.* 32(4): 684–91.

Speth, J. and Spielmann, K. "Energy Source, Protein Metabolism, and Hunter-gatherer Subsistence Strategies." *Journal of Anthropological Archaeology* 1983:2(1) 1–31.

US Senate Select Committee on Nutrition and Human Needs. 1977. *Dietary Goals for the United States. 2nd edition.* Washington (DC): US Government Printing Office.

Western Kentucky University. "Carbohydrates." Retrieved on 01 July 2013 from http://bioweb.wku. edu/courses/BIOL115/Wyatt/Biochem/Carbos.htm.

Wurtman, JJ. 1984. "The involvement of brain serotonin in excessive carbohydrate snacking by obese carbohydrate cravers." *J Am Diet Assoc.* 1984 Sep;84(9):1004-7. Review.

Wurtman RJ & Wurtman JJ. 1995. "Brain serotonin, carbohydrate-craving, obesity and depression." *Obes Res.* 1995 Nov;3 Suppl 4:477S–480S.

Young, C.M., Ringler, I., Greer, B.J. 1953 "Reducing and Post-Reducing Maintenance on the Moderate Fat Diet: Metabolic Studies." *Journal of the American Dietetic Association.* 29(9): 890–96.

acknowledgments

I would like to thank Louise Hay, a true visionary committed to bringing a wealth of information to those all around the world. You have transformed so many lives and are truly an inspiration. It is an honor to be published by you.

A huge, heartfelt thank you to the wonderful Hay House Team: Shannon Littrell, Stacey Smith, Margarete Nielsen, Christy Salinas, Charles McStravick, Lindsay McGinty, John Thompson, Patricia Lopez, Gail Gonzales, Tiffini Alberto, Heather Tate, Arron Alexis, Nicolette Salamanca, and most especially to my dear friend Reid Tracy for making this project come to life. Thank for your immense belief in this project and your work to impact people's lives on a worldwide scale.

I owe particular gratitude to my amazing team, as without them, nothing would be possible. To Kristin Penne, for keeping us all organized, on time, and sane. Your assistance means so much. To Oliver Stephenson, for your direction and support, I couldn't do it without you. You truly know how to apply your incredible commitment and talent to our mission. You make it all run! Thank you, also, for the beautiful photographs. And to Marianne McGinnis, without your hard work and dedication, this book would not exist. Your attention to detail and incredible research were invaluable, and you have made this book what it is. Your hard work and incredible talent were irreplaceable to this project; I can't thank you all enough for your dedication and commitment to creating outstanding content.

A very special thank you to my invaluable circle of experts: Gary Taubes, Dr. Robert Lustig, Dr. Mehmet Oz, Dr. Perricone, Dr. Northrup, Dr. David Ludwig, and Michael Pollan. And to Dr. Andrew Weil, thank you for your constant support and feedback.

To my JorgeCruise.com clients—your support in helping me refine this program, offering your comments, tips, and the courage to change your own lives have been a gift—thank you. You all inspire me each and every day.

To my 73,000 female *Costco Connection* clients who took the weight-loss challenge—your success with this plan was the true kickoff to our Happy Hormones, Slim Belly™ revolution, and I am so proud of you all. Thank you for your commitment and willingness to share your incredible stories.

To Ginnie Roeglin, Tim Talevich, and the rest of the *Costco Connection* team— thank you all so much for your continued support. Being able to work with your team is a true honor. With your help, we have changed so many lives, and I look forward to changing even more.

I wish to thank so many others who have contributed to this book as well as my overall vision and mission. Their advice, knowledge, and support have been so valuable and I would not be where I am today without them. While the list could go on and on, I wish to thank a few of them here, in alphabetical order.

Abra Potkin	Bobby Flay	Diane Sawyer
Al Roker	Bruce Barlean	Eben Pagan
Alexandra Cohen	Carol Brooks	Frank Kern
Anthony Robbins	Cathy Chermol	Hanna Richert
Bill Geddie	Chef Art Smith	Howard Bragman
Bob Wietrak	Chef Emeril Lagasse	Jacqui Stafford
Bobbi Brown	Daniel Sheldon	Jairek Robbins

Janet Annino	Maggie Jaqua	Richard Heller
Jay Robb	Mario Batali	Robin Meade
Joanna Parides	Mark Sisson	Robin Roberts
Joe Fusco	Marta Fox	Scott Eason
John Redmann	Martha Stewart	Stephen Steigler
Jon Davidson	Maura Wogan	Steve Harvey
Jose Pretlow	Mel Maurer	Susan Haber
Joseph Quesada	Michael Koenings	Sushupti Yalamanchili
Katie Couric	Michelle McGowen	Suzanne Somers
Kelly Ripa	Natalie Morales	Suze Orman
Lance Bass & the Dirty Pop Team @ SiriusXM Satellite Radio	Oprah Winfrey	Terence Noonan
	Pennie Ianniciello	Tim Austgen
Leslie Marcus	President Bill Clinton	Toni Richi
Linda Fennell	Rachael Ray	Travis Rosser
Lisa Gregorisch-Dempsey	Richard Galanti	Wayne Dyer

about the author

JORGE CRUISE is the #1 *New York Times* best-selling author of 19 weight-loss books. His mission is to guarantee weight loss for busy people. Science has proven that fitness begins in the kitchen, not in the gym. By merging break-through dietary science with great taste, he produces belly-fat-melting menus.

He has appeared on numerous television shows, including the *Dr. Oz Show, The Rachael Ray Show, LIVE! with Kelly and Michael,* CNN, *Good Morning America,* the *Today* show, *Dateline NBC,* and *The View.* He is a contributor to *First for Women* magazine and *The Costco Connection* magazine.

CONNECT WITH JORGE SOCIALLY AT:

Facebook.com/JorgeCruise

YouTube.com/JorgeCruise

JorgeCruise.Tumblr.com

Instagram.com/JorgeCruise

Twitter.com/JorgeCruise

Pinterest.com/JorgeCruise

Plus.Google.com/105974062782773382937

FREE MENU FOR WOMEN OVER 40

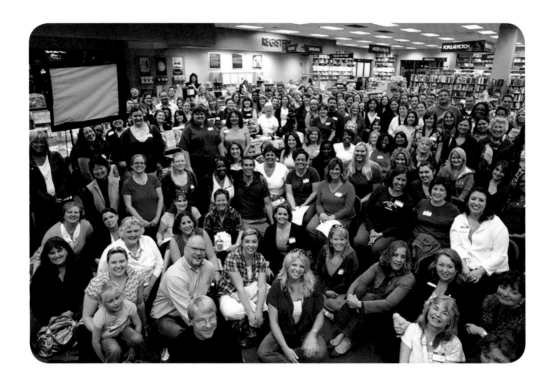

Go to JorgeCruise.com to join my FREE e-mail club
and get access to more menus and important information
such as reports, tips, videos, and more.

Visit HappyHormonesSlimBelly.com/FREE and join today!

We hope you enjoyed this Hay House book.
If you'd like to receive our online catalog featuring additional information
on Hay House books and products, or if you'd like to find out more
about the Hay Foundation, please contact:

Hay House, Inc., P.O. Box 5100, Carlsbad, CA 92018-5100
(760) 431-7695 or (800) 654-5126
(760) 431-6948 (fax) or (800) 650-5115 (fax)
www.hayhouse.com® • www.hayfoundation.org

Published and distributed in Australia by:
Hay House Australia Pty. Ltd., 18/36 Ralph St., Alexandria NSW 2015 •
Phone: 612-9669-4299 • *Fax:* 612-9669-4144 • www.hayhouse.com.au

Published and distributed in the United Kingdom by:
Hay House UK, Ltd., Astley House, 33 Notting Hill Gate, London W11 3JQ •
Phone: 44-20-3675-2450 • *Fax:* 44-20-3675-2451 • www.hayhouse.co.uk

Published and distributed in the Republic of South Africa by:
Hay House SA (Pty), Ltd., P.O. Box 990, Witkoppen 2068 •
Phone/Fax: 27-11-467-8904 • www.hayhouse.co.za

Published in India by:
Hay House Publishers India, Muskaan Complex, Plot No. 3, B-2, Vasant Kunj,
New Delhi 110 070 • *Phone:* 91-11-4176-1620 • *Fax:* 91-11-4176-1630 •
www.hayhouse.co.in

Distributed in Canada by:
Raincoast, 9050 Shaughnessy St., Vancouver, B.C. V6P 6E5 •
Phone: (604) 323-7100 • *Fax:* (604) 323-2600 • www.raincoast.com

TAKE YOUR SOUL ON A VACATION

Visit www.HealYourLife.com® to regroup, recharge,
and reconnect with your own magnificence.
Featuring blogs, mind-body-spirit news, and life-changing wisdom
from Louise Hay and friends.

Visit www.HealYourLife.com today!